Bright
Side Up

1/18

Bright Side Up

100 WAYS TO BE HAPPIER RIGHT NOW

AMY SPENCER

A Perigee Book

A PERIGEE BOOK
Published by the Penguin Group
Penguin Group (USA) Inc.
375 Hudson Street, New York, New York 10014, USA
Penguin Group (Canada), 90 Eglinton Avenue East, Suite 700, Toronto,
Ontario M4P 2Y3, Canada
(a division of Pearson Penguin Canada Inc.)
Penguin Books Ltd., 80 Strand, London WC2R 0RL, England
Penguin Group Ireland, 25 St. Stephen's Green, Dublin 2, Ireland
(a division of Penguin Books Ltd.)
Penguin Group (Australia), 250 Camberwell Road, Camberwell, Victoria 3124, Australia
(a division of Pearson Australia Group Pty. Ltd.)
Penguin Books India Pvt. Ltd., 11 Community Centre, Panchsheel Park,
New Delhi—110 017, India
Penguin Group (NZ), 67 Apollo Drive, Rosedale, Auckland 0632, New Zealand
(a division of Pearson New Zealand Ltd.)
Penguin Books (South Africa) (Pty.) Ltd., 24 Sturdee Avenue, Rosebank, Johannesburg 2196,
South Africa

Penguin Books Ltd., Registered Offices: 80 Strand, London WC2R 0RL, England

While the author has made every effort to provide accurate telephone numbers and
Internet addresses at the time of publication, neither the publisher nor the author assumes
any responsibility for errors or for changes that occur after publication. Further, the
publisher does not have any control over and does not assume any responsibility for
author or third-party websites or their content.

Copyright © 2012 by Amy Spencer
Text design by Tiffany Estreicher

First edition: February 2012

Library of Congress Cataloging-in-Publication Data

Spencer, Amy, 1971–
   Bright side up : 100 ways to be happier right now / Amy Spencer.
      p.   cm.
   ISBN 978-0-399-53727-1
   1. Positive psychology.   2. Optimism.   3. Happiness.   I. Title.
   BF204.6.S74 2011
   158.1—dc23   2011036237

PRINTED IN THE UNITED STATES OF AMERICA

10   9   8   7   6   5   4   3   2

Most Perigee books are available at special quantity discounts for bulk purchases for sales
promotions, premiums, fund-raising, or educational use. Special books, or book excerpts,
can also be created to fit specific needs. For details, write: Special Markets, Penguin Group
(USA) Inc., 375 Hudson Street, New York, New York 10014.

To my family
Mom, Dad, and Liz
for being the huggy,
supportive kind.

CONTENTS

Contents

When Your CAREER Isn't Going Your Way . . .

When Your RELATIONSHIPS Could Use a Reboot . . .

When Your SOCIAL LIFE Goes a Little Awry . . .

When FAMILY AND FRIENDS Are Stressing You Out . . .

When TECHNOLOGY Is Breaking Down . . .

When You Hit a Bump in Your TRAVELS . . .

INTRODUCTION

What Does It Mean to See Bright Side Up?

A friend of mine performed a card trick for a group of us after dinner. It was one of those "Pick your card, I'll shuffle them, and . . . Oh, look, here it is, impossibly faceup in the middle of the deck!" He did the trick three times in a row and I still, for the life of me, couldn't see the solution. He being a close friend and me not wanting that slice of cheesecake much anyway, he taught me his secret: All it really involved was a quick flip of his fingers in the first cut of the deck and a good dose of performance from there. Really, I've thought since, it's like life: Like a magician practices his sleight of hand, we have the power to practice our sleight of mind. Like the card that appeared faceup in my friend's deck, we can all master turning the bright side faceup in our lives.

Seeing bright side up is just that: a way to look at life that makes it easier than ever to see the secret, to find the good. The way a magician can lead you to look at his hands from a different angle, we can look at our lives in a fresh way, turning mountains into molehills, our fury into calm, our irritation into gratification, and our anger lines into laughs.

Do you know those optical illusions that show two images at the same time? You instantly see one image right away, but it's a bit of a challenge to see the other: Is it a duck or a rabbit? Is it a couple kissing or a vase? Is it an assortment of black blocks or a word in white? Well, it's both. Just like life. There is always both. There is no right or wrong way to see something— but there are different ways.

Of course, we all have unique experiences in life, and some people struggle through much harder times than others. In my dimmer downtimes, I've been fired from jobs, rejected from others. I've done physical therapy, worn crutches and casts, had three broken bones and a big broken heart. I've had deaths in my family, deaths of my friends, and I sobbed myself into another state of being over the death of my cat. I've lost money, lost friends, lost faith; I've been robbed of my belongings and robbed of my dignity. I've been banged up on a bike and run down by a truck, had car accidents and miscarriages. Like many New Yorkers, I saw my city bombed and burned from the roof of my building and have watched my country struggle to stand tall again ever since. And now, each and every day, I work to keep my marriage strong, the paychecks coming, my friendships fed, the bills paid.

Some days, life makes it easy for us. The sun shines, the

work flows, the roads open, the love dotes, and the day unfolds before us like a red carpet. On days like that, it's easy to feel optimistic, right? The positivity flows like wine and we're tipsy with happiness. And then sometimes . . . well. Sometimes we hit barriers of bills, traffic, arguments, and tears. These are the days you need your optimism more than ever, when you're stuck in a rough moment and smiling is the last thing on your mind. This book is for *those* times. When your car battery dies, your child breaks a tooth, your flight gets canceled, and your relationship fails, seeing your situation from a new angle can change your experience for the better.

We now know, based on studies in optimism and happiness as well as recent developments in neuroscience and positive psychology, that while we can't always change what happens to us, we can change how we *see and feel* about what happens to us. And this is huge. Because it means that **you don't have to completely change your life to be happier—you just need to change how you see your life to be happier.**

And seeing your life half full doesn't just shape your state of mind. Research shows if you're optimistic, you're likely to live longer, have lower blood pressure, less chance of heart disease, a stronger immune system, and you tend to endure pain better. If you're an optimistic athlete, you win more games; if you're an optimistic politician, you win more elections; if you're an optimistic salesperson, you sell more products. And career optimism can lead to more job offers, faster promotions, and higher salaries as optimists are more likely to take risks, problem solve, and adapt to get the job done. And all of this stems from the idea that it's not necessarily what happens to you but how you see what happens to you that makes the difference. It is your perspective that changes what you experience and how happy you feel.

Every day has a blue sky, remember. Even the gray ones. You just can't always see the sun above the clouds. But if you could get a new perspective—if you could get inside a plane that passes through the clouds—well, there's your blue sky and sunny day that was there all along. The entries in this book are seats on that airplane, the other side of that optical illusion, and a new perspective for when you need it most. Read them from cover to cover, or just dip into the book every now and then for a quick pick-me-up or when you need a dose of emergency optimism during a tough day.

You may, like me, be terrible at flipping cards over at a cocktail party, but the more often you see the bright side of life faceup, the more you'll do it naturally, and the happier you'll become. Let me explain.

. . . .

The science of seeing it.

. . . .

You can create a "brighter" brain.

Let's say you're sitting at a café outdoors, enjoying lunch with some friends. When the bill comes you instinctively reach for your wallet and find . . . nothing. You check another pocket and still . . . nothing. Your wallet. *It's gone.* And what happens from here is what can change your experience, for *you* have the power to decide what it is. The key is in your brain.

You'll react to your lost wallet first on an unconscious level in your brain stem, the oldest part of the brain, also sometimes called the reptilian brain. This area runs the building: your breathing, heartbeat, and just in case, your internal alarm system. It's the part of your brain that sends that awful chill of panic through your body about your wallet—all warm and shivery at the same time—before you've even formed an emotional reaction to what's happened.

The moment then moves to the next oldest part of your brain, the so-called mammalian brain that houses your limbic system, or emotional brain. It is here that you unconsciously feel flashes of emotions: Maybe it's fear or panic or fright or uncertainty; at this level of the brain, you're not putting words to your feelings, you're just receiving a flood of emotion.

Finally, the lost wallet hits the outermost layer of your brain that was developed most recently, about seventy million years ago (ah, it feels like just yesterday). This layer is known as the cortex, and it's the part of our brain that does our thinking, reviewing, analyzing, and planning. It is here that your consciousness about your wallet takes hold and here that you'll put words to your feelings. *Oh my God*, you're now thinking. *What happened? Where is it? I'm freaking out.* And, eventually, as you come to accept that your wallet is gone, *Now what?*

The "Now what?" is where this book comes in. The "Now what?" is where you can practice seeing bright side up. The

"Now what?" is where you can process what's happened, analyze how it's making you feel, and review all your options of how to deal with it. And here's the cool part: By regularly responding to the "Now what?" systems of your brain bright side up, you can train your brain to react positively with less and less prompting. Yes, *train* it.

According to still-recent neuroscientific research, the brain is capable of "neuroplasticity," which means we can mold and change how it functions over time just like warm clay. By challenging yourself through "metacognition"—or thinking *about* your thinking—you can rewire the neurocircuitry in your brain so your go-to mind-set is a more positive one. Rather than reacting to the lost wallets of life with, *Now everything's ruined!* you can get better at thinking, *At least I enjoyed a nice lunch first* instead. The more you use those positive neural pathways in your brain, the more you'll start to react more positively naturally.

This means that if you want to be happier, you can be, *right now*. **You don't need a change in your life to make it what you want it to be. You simply need to change how you *see* your life to make it what you want it to be. You can live "the good life" with the very same life you have right now.** You don't need to make more money, or have a better kitchen, or drive a nicer car, or get a big promotion, or spend three weeks in Hawaii to be happy. By learning to see the more positive side of your everyday situations, you will learn to find happiness in what you already have around you. If you are enjoying the *experience* of your life, you will be happy.

The magic is in your experience.

You know how two people can have the same conversation and both walk away feeling something different? That's because it's not necessarily what is physically happening to us at the moment, but how we experience what is happening that makes the difference. How we engage ourselves and how we subjectively feel about an event determines what we take from it and how happy we are.

Who's to say who's happier? No one. You can't. "What we *can* say," writes psychologist Daniel Gilbert in his book *Stumbling on Happiness*, "is that all claims of happiness are claims from someone's *point of view*—from the perspective of a single human being whose unique collection of past experiences serves as a context, a lens, a background for her evaluation of her current experience." If you've never felt a single pain in your life, then a prick on your pointer finger is going to hurt. But ask a woman who's been through childbirth how that needle feels and—*pfft!*—she'll have a much different perspective. Tough times are relative, right? A flood in the basement seems like a big deal until you watch the devastating footage of the tsunami in Japan. A pebble in your shoe that makes it hard for you to walk isn't nearly as serious as a torn ligament that makes it nearly impossible to. But the ability to see the positive is not in direct proportion to how big or small the problem in front of you; it's based on how well you are able to shift your point of view.

So if you can shift all kinds of experiences in your life—

especially the bad and the ugly ones—into good, you'll end up feeling more positive about your life without necessarily changing a single "thing" around you. Seeing bright side up is not about belittling the bad things that happen to us; it's about learning to shift our perspective in the best way for each situation. And guess what: It's not always about feeling *bright*.

These strategies aren't about hanging rainbow posters and plastering on fake smiles when you're angry. It goes much deeper. Seeing bright side up is about achieving a level of happiness you can only reach in appreciation of *all* your life experiences, even if life doesn't feel very positive in the moment.

For example, a grueling bike ride uphill against the wind to surpass your personal best time is not going to feel good the whole way; sometimes, in fact, it'll feel so dreadful you'll wonder why you're putting yourself through it at all. But because the experience as a *whole* will make you feel healthy, strong, proud of yourself, and happy, it's a positive one. Relationships are the same way: They don't always feel good—especially those times your partner is doing that awful screechy thing with the fork on their plate—but the connection you're building on, working around, dancing with, and sustaining for a lifetime is what makes it a positive experience. **Every date doesn't lead to love, every week of hard work doesn't lead to success, and every car ride isn't full of green lights, but finding value and joy in the experience along the way is what makes the difference** between a life that feels full of roadblocks or full of joy. And the more you do it, the better.

Practice makes happy.

You've done this bright stuff before, of course. You know that time you gratefully kissed the ground after a rough flight? Or gave another driver the benefit of the doubt and let him merge in front of you? Or gasped at the beauty of a sunset? Those are ways of leaning toward the positive that make you feel better in the moment. And while some moments bring out the bright side instinctively—like sighing with relief that no one was cut on a piece of broken glass—sometimes it may not come as naturally. That's what this book is for: to provide new ways to find the positive. A card magician is always learning new techniques to fool our eye, right? Well, the more tricks we have in our arsenals, the better, too.

I'm not suggesting you instantly think happy in every moment. In fact, forcing it can actually be counterproductive, according to a 2003 study by Schooler, Ariely, and Loewenstein. In it, researchers had volunteers listen to Stravinsky's *Rite of Spring*—some of whom were told to try to consciously be happy while listening to it. Surprisingly, the participants who *tried* being happy actually felt worse. And if you've ever been commanded by a grocery store clerk to "Smile!" when she has no idea the day you're having or if you've been told by your friends to "Look on the bright side!" when you're still grieving a devastating loss, you know the feeling. But when you're sick and tired of *being* sick and tired, there are strategies for finding your way out of the gloom.

Take, for example, this email my mom just sent me about a water pipe that broke in my family home:

> We have owned this house for forty years, and we've had low water pressure from day one. For forty years we were careful not to flush the toilet or brush our teeth if someone was in the shower.
>
> This past fall we put in a new heating system, converting from oil to gas, which would greatly reduce our heating bill. During this construction process, a costly setback occurred: The water pipe from the street crumbled and broke at the entrance to the house while the plumbers were shutting off the water. We now had not only the expensive conversion, but had to pay for a major water pipe replacement that ran from the street to the house four feet underground. The end cost of that extra was about $3,000, which we had not anticipated. Oh well, we thought, that's life.
>
> However, it turned out to be a blessing in disguise. Not only do we have great water pressure now, but eventually the pipe would have broken anyway since it was so fragile. It could have broken when we were out of the house, or even on vacation. Imagine the basement flood if that happened! Or, can you also imagine, if it happened in the middle of a winter like this one where there was frozen earth and two to three feet of snow to dig through for a repair to be made? We were very, very lucky that it broke that day. Oh happy day!

I mean, gosh, can you see where I got *my* optimism? In that story alone, my parents are seeing bright side up in a number of ways. They recognize that life likes to uproot plans whether you like it or not (which we'll talk about in "See plans as just blueprints"); they see how lucky they are the pipe didn't break at a worse time (which we'll cover in "At least you're not . . ."); they're grateful for the joy of water pressure they haven't had in forty years (which we'll relate to in "Appreciate your abundance"); and knowing they'll soon be saving on their heating bills, they're excited for their future selves (a habit you'll learn about in "Put a bow on it for your future self").

I'm not saying that beneath all tragedy is great news, but **there is more than one way to look at a situation. The circumstances may not be within your control, but your perspective, attitude, and experience is *entirely* up to you.** If you focus on all the reasons your situation stinks, you will find plenty. And if you seek the benefits, you'll find those, too.

By learning how to spot and appreciate the small pleasures, your daily life can improve. If you aim to find the positive in any *glitch*uation—whether you're fixing a flat tire or returning a broken blender—you can make your experience feel like a better one.

A doctor may give you medicine and tell you to apply as needed, and these techniques are applicable for coping in many situations the very same way. When I suggest you "Rest for a minute . . . maybe two," that can help in your search for a relationship, your attempts at weight loss, while cleaning out your closet, or when you're brainstorming a business idea.

When I propose you "See life like a seesaw," that can work when you're stuck at a red light, leave a scarf behind, or lose a client. So use each idea as you see fit in your own life.

By giving you one hundred different ways to shift your perspective in gray situations, I hope to get your brain practicing in just the right way. The better you get at seeking out the bright sides on a regular basis, the faster it will become second nature. Before you know it, you'll be turning the bright on without even trying.

When You're Not Feeling Like Your Fantastic SELF . . .

Look, your life is art.

Last summer, I was having so much fun walking along the water at the beach, I took photos of my toes in the splashing surf. Yet when I looked at the cool shots later, the first thing I thought was, *Ugh, look at my cankles.*

Yep, I have cankles. Essentially, this means my calves hit my feet without slimming down into adorably skinny little ankles. My legs are more like, sorta, two tapered telephone poles. Of course, when I showed the pictures to my best friend Todd, he said, "What are you *talking* about? All I see is water and a cute foot." And that's when I realized I was being overly self-critical. And every time you overlook the good stuff because of a "flaw" you think you have, you are, too.

Unusual features and imperfections don't dampen things; they elevate them. Mistakes in a coin or stamp are what make them collector's items, worth far more than their face value. **You are art in just the same way. So figure out what your thing is and flaunt it.**

Edgar Degas painted the folds of flesh on robust women beautifully. Common quilts made by the women of Gee's Bend, Alabama, strayed so far from traditional patterns they've hung in the Whitney Museum. The Leaning Tower of Pisa might not have gotten a glance were it not for its unintentional angle. And Barbra Streisand and Lady Gaga prove that unique noses can help you stand out and shine.

Those little things we don't like about ourselves are just that: little things. So you have a cowlick, a mole, a waddle, a bulge, or a bald spot—big whoop! A little thing only becomes big when you set the magnifying glass in front of it. In fact, chances are those "flaws" are only obvious to you.

You are—and I know this to be true—a profoundly complex, interesting, wonderful, beautiful human being despite or perhaps because of all the small things that make you different. So figure out what makes you art and defend it. What's in you that isn't in everyone else? Whether you order your dessert before dinner or, like me, proudly get your money's worth at an all-you-can-eat Brazilian *churrascaria*, odd can be beautiful if you own it. But there is also beauty in what can seem ordinary, too. Just like NBC once promoted its television reruns as "new to you," what seems average in your eyes can be extraordinarily special to someone else. As artist Georgia O'Keeffe once said when she had an idea for a picture, "How ordinary. Why paint that old rock? Why not go for a walk instead? But then I realize that to someone else, it may not seem so ordinary."

What is boring to you—or odd, or imperfect, or unattractive—can be endearing to others the minute you choose to own it. Your life is art. Put a big frame around it and show it off. I have cankles. But they're my cankles on my legs and if I'm using them to kick up seawater on the sand, then that's a pretty great place for them to be.

Start looking at yourself from a larger place, too. In the big picture, you're perfectly balanced and miraculously wonderful. A priceless work of art.

....

Ask your
one-hundred-year-old self.

....

We all wonder which path to take, what career to pursue, who to marry, where to settle down, and when to retire. But you know who can answer that better than you? Your one-hundred-year-old self. When I'm torturing myself over which path to take, I imagine myself as an old, wise woman and ask her: "What should I do?" I ask the wrinkled, wise person I'll be blessed to become, sage in experience, a survivor of bad choices and missed chances, the one person who can look back on my life and see where I went wrong, got scared, or grew weak. Try it for yourself. Ask: What should I do?

Your one-hundred-year-old self will be gentle and kind, but it will also be the voice of conviction, strength, and fearlessness you might have forgotten you have inside you. It's that voice who'll say, "For Pete's sake, just kiss her already." And, "My goodness, if you're not going to walk in there and ask for the job, I'll ask *for* ya."

Your one-hundred-year-old self will tell you if you're wasting your time on busywork or with phony people instead of spending quality time with people who matter, and if you're overanalyzing emails in your relationship or fighting when you should be fixing. So if you're feeling down on your life, stuck in a rut, or worried about pursuing your dreams, imagine your older self rocking on your front porch, a lifetime of experiences and great loves behind you. When that person looks back at you, what advice might they give you now? I think they would be kind: "You are so *young*! Please, don't waste another day feeling bad about your life. If you only *knew* the great things around the corner for you. The love, the success, the pride that you'll feel in yourself for pursuing what your heart wants. Please don't let that big spirit and big talent go to waste. Go on, follow your heart and *live your life*."

When I got engaged to my husband, Gustavo, my dad filmed my then-ninety-year-old Gramma Ruth giving us marriage advice. "With Howard and I, I was the meek one, and so whatever he said, I went along with," Gramma told us. "And it wasn't until he died that I decided I had to come out and be myself and speak up. So speak up!"

Your one-hundred-year-old self might do the same for you when you're scared about new things. Whether you need courage, confidence, or a dose of tough love, the view from up ahead can help. "Are you kiddin' me?" your older self might say. "Of course you don't know what will happen next, but if you don't try, you'll never know. And then I'll be stuck rocking in this darn chair the last decade of my life wondering, 'What if?' Don't do that to me, kid. Take the chance already and see what happens." Your own wise old soul will help you put things into perspective. Just ask.

Flip-flop it.

My friend Monchi, from Panama, was planning a party with his housemate Mariana. They wanted to throw an upscale party at their recently renovated home, but Mariana had just had her wood floors redone, and she didn't want people putting pockmarks into the fresh finish with their high heels.

"It's tacky to ask people to take their shoes off inside, right?" he asked.

"Right," she said. "But it's also tacky to say they're not allowed inside at all."

Then she stumbled upon the perfect solution: "We'll throw a chancletini party!"

"A *what*?" asked Monchi.

"*Chancletas* and martinis!"

In Panama, the word *chancleta* means "flip-flop" (that is, those rubber beach shoes), so at this party, they'd serve martinis to guests wearing flip-flops all night long.

Well, people went nuts for it. They went on *chancleta* shopping trips, buying wacky pairs decorated with wild colors, big plastic flowers, or superheroes from the ninety-nine-cent store. The first thing people did when they walked in the room was point at one another's feet and whoop with laughter.

"Half the photos people took at the party were of peoples' feet!" said Monchi.

Guests loved it *so* much they're asking for Chancletini II—and all of this sprouted from Mariana's fear that her floors would be mussed. The party hosts took what seemed like a negative request and flipped it into something positive, surprising, and delightful.

The lesson? **There is always another way to look at things, a solution for handling something by making a different physical, mental, or emotional choice.** Think about that the next time you find yourself in a mental pickle: *Is there another angle to this? Should I come at this from the other side?* Singleness, for instance, is also freedom. Loneliness is also time to think. Frustration at work is also passion: You wouldn't feel this bad if you didn't want it so much. Pull a page from Monchi and Mariana's chancletini party and flip-flop your next problem.

If you're broke and still want to celebrate your birthday, have a cereal party. If you've ripped a gash in your favorite jeans, stitch them up with bright green thread. Flipping it can take the thing you're most scared of, embarrassed about, or leery to express and make it more memorable than ever.

Just after my friend, actress and author Diane Farr, had sent out a big batch of engagement cards reading "Engaged!" to her friends and family, she found out her husband-to-be was a louse and called off the wedding. Embarrassed by the cute cards she'd sent out and unsure of how to notify people without wanting to crawl under a rock, she embraced the very cards themselves and flipped them: A week later, she sent out identically designed cards that read, this time, "Single! Picked the wrong guy. Gave him the wrong finger. Thanks for your support." The laughs led to heaping support from her loved ones, an appearance on *Oprah*, and a chance to meet the right guy for her, with whom she's now raising their three beautiful kids. See how she did it? Pick the worst part of your situation and build up just that.

No matter what life doles out, we have the ability to turn the very worst into the very best. So kick off your shoes and free up your mind. If you're feeling like a flop, flip it.

Steer life like a motorcycle.

My sister, Liz, took a weekend course to get her motorcycle license and kept getting confused about which way she was supposed lean to get the bike around some orange cones in the parking lot. Her instructor, seeing that she was struggling, said there was a golden rule of riding: "Look where you want to go and the bike will steer you straight to it." What a great rule for living, too: **Look where you want to go and life will steer you straight to it.**

Life draws us where we're looking; if you want to be in the career or relationship or other life situation of your dreams, focus on where you want to go. It's when you don't have a vision of where you're heading that you will get lost.

I spoke with maze designer Adrian Fisher of Dorset, England, famous for creating life-size hedge mazes, mirror mazes, and corn mazes. He said one of his tricks is to confuse people with what he calls "the motorway effect," in which we underestimate a turn we've taken. It's like when you're driving on a freeway, Fisher told me, "and the whole road bends to the left for a mile and a half. You'll think you're still going north, but you're now facing a bit south of west. You'd be surprised," he says. "The motorway effect is one of the ways that, as a maze designer, I deceive people. When they gradually go around a curve, I quietly wind them up. And I often succeed in detaching them from their assumed reference point."

The motorway effect happens in life, too. A woman I know has been talking for years about the family she wants to have, and yet she keeps dating international charmers who only pop into town once a month to take her out for fine meals with famous people; distracted by the glamorous life, she forgets to focus on what she really wants. And a man I know used to talk about spending a year in Europe while he was young and hungry, after sticking out his dull office job a little longer. It's been fourteen years and he's still at the same job, older and pretty well fed by now. It's the motorway effect: Distracted by the perks of stability, he barely noticed his dream falling further behind in the rearview mirror. But as any good GPS will remind you, it's *never* too late to redirect.

Do you want to avoid the motorway effect? Try what my mom, a couples therapist, taught me fifteen years ago while I was working as a social worker for foster children in New York. Driving together one day, I told her how I wasn't sure I wanted to stay in the field, but I didn't know what to do instead.

"Tell me this," she said. "If you could paint a picture of your future life, what would you want your home to look like?"

I described a place on the water with an office on the second story overlooking the view, and how I wrote for a living when I wasn't playing with my husband and kids.

"Now," she said, "every time you hit a fork and have a choice to make in life, think of that picture and take the path that leads you closer to it."

Fifteen years later, I'm getting there. I'm only in a single-story house that's a good six blocks from the ocean, but I do write for a living while my husband paints in the other room. And the kid thing? We've been working on that. As my sister did with her motorcycle, I've looked where I've wanted to go, and life has helped steer me toward it. Do this for yourself. Give yourself a picture to steer toward.

If you could paint the perfect picture of your future life, what would *your* home look like? How would you feel going shopping, taking a walk, talking to neighbors? Would you have a partner in your life, and if so, how would you treat each other and feel with one another? What do you spend your free time doing? What's the view out of your kitchen window? How will you feel when you wake up in the morning, and how will you spend your day? From now on, every time you hit a fork and have a choice to make in life, take the path that leads you closer to *that* picture.

By giving yourself a clear picture to steer toward, you'll avoid being misled by a motorway effect. Give yourself the gift of a clear vision on who you want to be, how you want to feel, and then set your course to hit your mark. Steer life like you would a motorcycle. Look where you want to go, and life will get you there. Just do me a favor, please. Wear a helmet.

Take pride in persistence.

Our culture rewards quick thinking: We communicate in 140 characters or less, get our news from headlines, watch marriages split up before the first anniversary cake is defrosted, and lease cars we'll return before they've even lost that "new car smell." So it's natural for us to pick up projects, relationships, and hobbies like disposable razors. But to have the willpower to stick with something? To actually focus and devote yourself to a passion long enough to learn from it? *That's* worth celebrating.

Sometimes it's not how perfect the job you're doing is; it's that you're doing it. **Quantity gets a bad rap against quality, but when you're exhausted by the hours you've invested in something that's taking longer than you thought, be darn proud of the quantity.** As minister James Watkins once said, "A river cuts through rock, not because of its power, but because of its persistence." And I saw the power of persistence for myself watching my dad, who not only makes his own telescopes for fun but one year ground his own mirror to put in one.

"It takes a tremendous amount of patience," my dad said as he explained the process of grinding and polishing glass into a mirror perfect enough to capture the light from a star sixteen light-years from Earth. It began with two six-inch glass disks he sprinkled with Carborundum abrasive and water and rubbed together by hand until the top disk became concave, like a makeup mirror, so it would magnify. "That's the easy part," he says. Yeah, an easy part that takes about forty hours; all in all, a six-inch mirror takes about eighty hours to make.

But when he put his handmade mirror into his telescope for the first time, he was blown away. "The moon craters were so sharp," he says. "It is impossible to describe the feeling of looking through a telescope at a cluster of stars and realize you fashioned it from your own hands. I just thought, *I can't believe I made this in my basement.*"

Now, that's some dogged persistence that yielded a tangible payoff. But how do you know if your persistence is paying off? First, ask yourself: "How much have I learned about the process?" Maybe your herb garden isn't thriving, but how much more do you know about planting than the day you dropped in your first seed? Maybe your marriage seems shaky at times, but how much more do you know about balance and sacrifice than you did on your very first date? If you've learned anything at all, it has been worth it. And even if what you've learned is that it's time for you to put down the shovel or concede a loss or walk away, *that's* an invaluable lesson.

Second, ask yourself this: "Have others quit where I have persevered?" As author Malcolm Gladwell notes in his book *Outliers*, based on research led by psychologist K. Anders Ericsson, one measure of aptitude lies in how many hours you've invested in practice—and for greats like Bill Gates and the Beatles, it's ten thousand. Ten *thousand* hours. So if you haven't spent that much time yet on the cause, well, forgive yourself for not being the Beatles. And congratulate yourself for having the gumption to have kept going! Failure is everywhere: One in four restaurants fail in their first year. And far more than that many marriages do. "I've missed more than nine thousand shots in my career," noted NBA legend Michael Jordan in a powerful Nike commercial. "I've lost almost three hundred games. Twenty-six times I've been trusted to take the game-winning shot . . . and missed. I have failed over and over and over again in my life. And that is why I succeed."

Sometimes, devotion counts. So look at the effort you've put in and all you've learned until now, and be proud of how far you've carried through.

Live ten minutes in the life of "the ideal you."

My friend Ben once told me, "The ideal number of martinis is the same as grilled cheese: one and a half. One just isn't enough, but two is pushing it. Stick with one and a half and you can't go wrong." And my ideal self agrees. But when I have either a martini or a grilled cheese in front of me—both at the same time seems like an unfair slice of heaven, really—I'm hard-pressed to listen. Because there's the "I" we are, and there's the ideal "I" we *wish* we were. And very often, there's a big space in between.

Maybe the ideal you has a cup of hot green tea in a comfy chair by the window in the early morning light, while the real you puts on coffee while brushing your teeth and checking emails in the dark because, well, you don't have a comfy chair by a window.

Maybe the ideal you winds down at the end of the day reading one of the greatest novels of the twentieth century while listening to *Tosca*, while the real you curls up under a blanket on the couch for three mind-numbing hours of TiVo.

Maybe the ideal you throws weekly dinner parties with Ina Garten recipes paired with fine wine, while the real you is so tired by Friday, you only have time to doctor up some jarred pasta sauce paired with a bottle of Two-Buck Chuck.

We know that living as our ideal selves makes us feel better.

But this is real life we're talking about, a vortex of urgent emails and work deadlines, carpools and tax appointments, and marathons of TV shows you simply can't tear yourself away from (ahem, cooking competition shows). So not only do we forget how important it is to allow ourselves a chance to *be* the person we wish we were, we don't have the time!

Well, you do. Kind of. Because you don't need as much time as you think. **Spending just ten minutes a day feeding those dreams of your ideal self will bring you closer to feeling as if you were living it every second.**

Maybe you don't have time to train for an Ironman, till an organic garden, learn Italian, and refurbish old furniture while working a full-time job and dreaming about a pied-à-terre in Paris. But you *can* spend ten minutes planting sage in the kitchen window. You *can* read eight pages of a great book. You *can* go for a brisk walk around the block before you get back to work. And just those ten minutes of living your ideal life will fill you with such bursts of pride and productivity that you'll want to do so much more.

It's not practical to believe we'll make all the right food choices, spend all the right money, and read all the right books all the time. So we shouldn't beat ourselves up when we don't. Not only are we being unfair to ourselves to feel like failures if we don't meet all of our own ideal expectations, but reaching the pinnacle of our perfect selves would leave no room for dreams! Instead, give yourself a goal you have no excuse to miss: Every day, for just ten minutes, do *one small thing* that your ideal self would do. It will feel like clicking the "on" switch of a happy life, setting the scene for you to fulfill more of the best self you want to and know you can be.

Always spring for your limo.

When I spoke to young Grammy-winning country star Miranda Lambert as she got her hair and makeup done for a photo shoot for *Redbook* magazine, she talked about something Reba McEntire told her. "Always show up like a star," she said Reba told her. "Always spring for that limo. If you appear like a star, people will treat you like that and you *will* be one."

I think Reba's onto something. In your own unique way in your own unique moment, always spring for "the limo" in your own life—whatever it is that physically expresses who you want to be, from a loving partner to a serious businessperson. You can thank the psychological gift of "embodied cognition" for how this helps you feel like and become just what you want. "Our thoughts and our attitudes show up in our bodies, and what your body is doing affects your attitude," explains neuropsychologist Rick Hanson, author of *Buddha's Brain: The Practical Neuroscience of Happiness, Love, and Wisdom.*

For example, Hanson told me, if you tend to feel you hold back in conversation, physically leaning into the conversation can change how the conversation goes. If you're overwhelmed by life and feeling weak, lifting up your chest in a stance of strength can alter how you approach it. "Adopt the posture, and that will encourage you to adopt the feelings and attitudes that will follow," says Hanson. "If you form a vision of the life you want in some important way, and you see yourself in that vision as *already having it*, that pulls you into the stance, the facial expression, and the look that brings the sense of already being that way. And it sends all kind of subliminal messages to others that you *are* what you want." The way you feel and express yourself can make you the most confident person in the room or the most self-defeating—and that relative status is a big determinant in the events that follow. When I got my first editing job at a magazine, for example, I was wary about my role until my business cards came in. Each time I handed out a card, I was bolstered by the word "editor" under my name, which made me adopt the physical posture of an editor, which led me to be treated like one.

So how do you know what the limo is for your particular need? Picture someone who *has* what you want and ask yourself: *What are they doing, how are they acting, or what are they portraying that I can, too?* If you want to be a loving partner, do what looks like loving and you will become and be treated as someone who is. If you want to be taken seriously at work, wear the smart outfit one of your bosses might wear, and you'll start to be treated the same way.

Use embodied cognition to your advantage in all areas of your life. If you're feeling beat down or undeserving or unspecial, your energy and body language will express that you feel that way, and you'll be treated that way. Instead, **spring for your limo. Put on the costume or posture of who you want**

to be. Fake it until you make it. Physically act like the person you *wish* you were and your limo will take you straight there.

Take the microphone.

It was over a decade ago that I walked into a mattress dealership on a rainy day, gullibly gushed over their "rainy day sale," and put down a "fully refundable" cash deposit to hold the deal on a mattress. I also gave them my home address in case I chose to purchase it. Yet the next morning, I answered the doorbell to see two men holding that very mattress!

Furious, I marched back to the store to ask for my money. "Your deposit is no longer refundable," said the salesman, citing a loophole in which I didn't provide the proper line of refusal. And after fifteen minutes making every argument I could think of, I asked to see a manager.

"I *am* the manager," he said. I should have known. I was shaking in anger and wished I had more chutzpah. But as he stood up and smiled charmingly at a couple who'd just walked in, I simply decided I *did*.

"I am not walking out of here without my deposit," I said as he strolled past me.

"That's fine," he said with a smirk, "stay as long as you like."

Just then, a strange feeling bubbled up from my nonconfrontational belly, and I turned to the room of customers and shouted like a girl on a soapbox.

"Don't trust this man!" I yelled. "He'll try to convince you to put down a deposit, and then he'll take it from you! I know I sound crazy," I shouted (oh, and I did; I sounded *crazy*), "but he'll charm you and he'll steal from you. Do *not* give him cash, do *not*—"

"Okay, *okay*," the salesman said, scurrying back. I walked out with my cash in hand.

It was a surreal experience, but it gave me a rush, because when we feel we're not getting what we deserve, it's our job to speak up. The truth is, though, I don't do it often enough. As irritated as I sometimes get by "the principle of the thing," I look at the hours involved in getting that fee removed, that rule changed, that order switched, and I wave it off. Apathy-R-Us. But what surprises me more is how often we're *asked* what we want and still don't speak up—as if someone has handed us the microphone and we still don't say a word.

One night, for instance, my mom ordered crab cakes at a restaurant, took one bite, and said, "These taste like dishwater." We thought she'd tell the server, but she shrugged.

"That's all right," she said, putting down her fork. "It's fine."

We reminded her she was paying her hard-earned money for what tasted like greasy dishes—*so* not fine. So when the server came back and asked how we were, she spoke up and got a different meal.

We humans are not mind readers. Sure, we can read body language and expressions in the eyes of others. But we cannot read minds—not at work, not at play, not in love. So if you want flowers, or a phone call, or time for yourself the first ten minutes after you walk in the door from work, take the microphone and speak your piece.

If you want it, say you want it. If it's not fine, say it's not fine. If you're looking for something serious, say, "I'm looking for something serious." And if it's high up on your "Important to Me" list, speak up and *say* so.

Ask for what you want in life, speak what's on your mind. You don't need a megaphone in a mattress store, but when someone asks what you want, answer honestly. Your voice deserves to be heard.

....

Rephrase to reframe.

....

When you go for a job interview, there's always one sticky question in the bunch. It's the kind you wish you could answer with, "I get lazy on Friday afternoons and I thought my boss was an arrogant jerk . . . why do you ask?" But you'd never say those things, really. Instead, you spin a brighter version. And though that means focusing on just one way to look at it, you're still expressing a truth that keeps the interview packaged in a positive light.

It works in job interviews and it works in life: If you want to see things in a more positive light, frame it and *phrase* it in a more positive way. Maybe you can frame a lousy day as challenging, recognize that a selfish person helps you practice your patience, and surmise that a tasteless burrito could've had more flavor. And if you hated a movie? Well, maybe you just didn't *love* it. I'm not suggesting you say you've liked what you haven't and loved days that brought you down; what I am suggesting is you find a way to rephrase bad moments so you, in turn, will feel better about it. You have this skill already: It's the one you use when you're opening a gift from Aunt Flora ("It looks so . . . warm!") or telling your friend what you thought of his performance ("I . . . couldn't stop watching!"). Use it in your own life, for yourself. Rephrase the bad moments in order to reframe them.

One way to think about it begins with what Martin Seligman, PhD, a pioneer in the field known as Positive Psychology, calls your "explanatory style." How you explain a setback can make all the difference in what you take away from it. Pessimists, he says, will judge a bad situation as personal, pervasive, and permanent, while an optimist sees it as impersonal, specific, and temporary. Say, for example, Mary and Kim both lose their jobs in the same office on the same day for the same stated reason: cutbacks. Mary is gutted, as she sees this as a *personal* insult to her capabilities and something future employers are *all* going to agree with, which is why she's *never* going to find another good job again. Kim, on the other hand, feels it's *not personal*, it's just some bad luck; and if she could have this *one* job, she'll *surely* get another. Two people, one misfortune, two future paths forged. Now: Who would you rather interview for a new position?

Lighter language can also affect your motivation. Recently, for instance, I was telling Gus about a workday I was dreading. "This week has been a nightmare," I said, "and I have another hellish day ahead." Then I heard the words I was using and stopped myself short. *Nightmare?* I thought. *Really?* I mean compared to soldiers fighting through sandstorms in firelike heat with their lives on the line, I was just *typing* for ten hours; it wasn't anything close to "hell" at all. Hearing how I was talking about it helped me reframe what was ahead and reflect what it really was: a difficult workday I'd soon get through.

Using positive language for a negative experience may be stretching it some, but there *is* a brighter truth if you choose to focus on it. In fact, why not start a neutral conversation talking about positive things, too? When you're meeting someone new, instead of groaning about work, ask about their *favorite* movie, the *best* meal they've ever had, and their *coolest* vacation. Set a positive tone and see what develops.

Try it. Use more constructive words for a day and see how you feel. Because if you want to focus on how lousy a day has been, you'll most likely feel that way yourself; but if you say it just wasn't your favorite day of the week, it won't seem so bad. It may even seem, dare you say, a little bit *good*.

Do the can-can.

Two years ago, I miscarried my first pregnancy at eleven weeks. But in an effort to find control during a sad stage when I felt I had none, I began getting acupuncture to balance my health and up my odds for the next time. One of the things my acupuncturist suggested was a food plan that wasn't for the weak: No caffeine. No dairy. No wheat. No alcohol. No refined grains. No cold drinks. No raw vegetables. Some terrible-tasting teas. And a gagging supplementation of spoonfuls of blackstrap molasses I had to pinch my nose to get down.

The next week, I went in on the verge of tears.

"How's it going?" she asked.

"It's fine," I said. "I mean . . . I hate it! I just don't know how to eat anymore." My voice quivered as I explained the walls I'd hit that week. I'd wanted a salad, but it was raw, so I thought I'd get a sandwich, but I couldn't have the bread. Pasta was out. Icy smoothies were out. "And when my husband got a slice of pizza," I said, "I couldn't have that, either—not even the 'salad' pizza with cooked veggies on top!"

My acupuncturist patiently nodded and then said this: "I'm hearing a lot about what you can't eat. What about what you *can*?"

Aargh. She was right. And I've since learned this is true of lots of things in our lives, especially in our health. It happens when a cholesterol issue keeps you from eating the steaks you love, an allergy issue takes gluten and your favorite pizza off the table, or when you blow out your knee and can't play basketball or run to the car. When our health suffers, it's natural for us to think about what we *can't* do, but we'll have an entirely different experience when we ask what we can. **Do the can-can. And marvel when you realize this: The list of what you *can* do is so much bigger than what you can't.**

If you focus on what you can't have, that is all you'll see—and every dieter knows how that works. The minute you eliminate certain foods, they're all you think about. And studies have shown that by trying "not" to think about things, it's exactly what you will. In 2007, when psychologist James Erskine, PhD, had participants taste and rate some chocolate, one group was asked to think about chocolate, one group was asked *not* to think about chocolate, and the third wasn't told anything about it. The result? The group instructed *not* to think about chocolate not only recorded more thoughts about chocolate, they ate more chocolate! The suppression of thoughts led to the exact opposite.

It's a law of the universe, really: What you give your attention to, you will attract. If you think you'll never get the job or won't be able to get your date to like you, you'll create such a negative energy within you, you'll probably prove yourself right. And like that chocolate study, if all you're thinking about is how you can't have Ring Dings and ice cream, beware the road that leads to 7-Eleven. From now on, turn your back on the restrictions and shift your attention to what's open.

Life has so much to offer. It's an endless bounty of things to see, do, eat, experience, and love. So the next time life becomes the buzzkill of the party by telling you what you can't do, focus on what you *can*. You'll be blown away by how much bigger that list is. So hit the dance floor and start kicking.

....

Keep your eyes on
your own paper.

....

You know about the Rumble in the Jungle, right? Here's how the boxing match between Muhammad Ali and world heavyweight champion George Foreman went down in 1974: Ali knew he didn't have the strength of his younger competitor—so instead of trying to be stronger, he used what *he* had: the ability to take a punch. He trained, essentially, in being pummeled. He *planned* on being beat for round after round, to be able to stand against the ropes in a "rope-a-dope" move while Foreman hit him. Ali knew that if he could take the pain, he could tire out Foreman and take back control. In the eighth round, against all odds, Ali knocked out Foreman to take the title.

The story reminds me of my grade school days, when a teacher strolling the aisles between our desks during a test would say, "Keep your eyes on your own paper." Those teachers were right. Instead of leaning over our desks to copy what our neighbors are writing, we should be writing our own stories and working off our own strengths, just like Ali.

It's wonderful advice when you find yourself feeling you're not as good as, or as smart as, or as *enough* as someone else. Because you're not someone else! Become content with who you are and what you were born on this earth to do. **Keep your eyes on your own paper and do what makes your life—your paper—the best it can be.**

If we keep our eyes on our own paper, we'll find the rope-a-dope move within us all. It's what also worked for Madonna: "I know I'm not the best singer and not the best dancer, but I'm not interested in that," she said in her 1991 tour documentary film *Truth or Dare*. "I'm interested in pushing people's buttons and being provocative and political." She was interested, in other words, in leveraging her strengths and using what she had plenty of: charisma, shock value, and smarts. And now, decades later, we consider the woman who didn't think she could sing to be one of the most influential singers of the century.

From now on, look at your life as the only one you need to focus on. Don't worry about the looks, the relationships, or the jobs other people have. Don't let the moms in the playgroup affect how you parent. Don't let the people watching affect how you dance. And don't let someone else's style change how you want to dress. Express yourself. Just look, love, work, and dance the best way *you* know how. Remember, we don't know someone's whole story just by sneaking a peek at his or her cover sheet. If all we're seeing is the good stuff, it's natural to be envious. But there's so much more we're not seeing. We don't know the past they carry with them, the troubles they've faced, the relationships they struggle with, the debts they have. As my wise sister-in-law, Mariana, said to me one day, "Anytime someone comes to me with a problem, I always tell them that if everyone in the world put their problems into a giant hole, they would probably end up picking out their own again."

Keep your eyes on your own paper. Write your own story.

Take whatever makes your soul soar in what you do, who you love, and how you want to feel, and pen your own happy ending.

Yes, go for a walk!

I was feeling lethargic one Saturday when I ran my options by my husband.

"Should I go for a power walk?" I asked him. (Yeah, that's right, people. I power walk. And I only care a little bit that I look funny doing it.) "Or," I proposed, "should I just, like, take a nap?"

"You should go for a walk," said Gus.

"*Should* I, though?" I asked. "I'm tired, so if I took a nap I'd be rested."

"But if you go for a walk," he said, "you'll wake up."

"You're right," I said. "I should." Then I lumbered toward the bedroom to pull on my sneakers. *"Or,"* I said, stopping halfway, "I could maybe just stretch out on the couch so . . . not an official nap, but just resting." I smiled. He smirked. "Right?" I said. "Wouldn't that be good?"

"You know what would be *good*," he said, "is that walk. It was *your* idea."

Foiled again, but for the better. Because when I came back from panting through my power walk, I felt alive. I was bursting with energy, brimming with pride, and thankful as all get out for a husband who wouldn't let me talk *him* into telling *me* it was okay to give in to my sloth.

I rationalize my way around in circles like this all the time, but I suspect I'm not alone. For if we're not running through a conversation like this with a spouse, friend, roommate, or otherwise, we're often having this conversation with *ourselves*. And here's what I've learned about it: If you're debating whether or not you should get up and out for a minute, the answer is almost always the same. Yes, go for a walk! Yes, take a stroll. Yes, get outside and get going!

We already know that going for a walk is healthy for your body: A study published in the *New England Journal of Medicine* in 1999, for example, showed that walking at a moderate pace for up to three hours a week can cut the risk of heart disease in women by as much as 40 percent. But walking can also alter your *mind*. In a study published in January 2011 in the *Proceedings of the National Academy of Sciences*, researchers found the hippocampus in the brain—an area vital to the formation of memories—can be strengthened by regular walking. Researchers sent one group of sedentary volunteers walking around a track three times a week for up to forty minutes, and had another partake in less aerobic activities like yoga. One year later, the brain scans of the walkers showed the hippocampus had increased in size by about 2 percent, while among the less aerobic exercisers, the same area decreased by 1.4 percent (which is about the average loss in adults each year).

But the best part of walking in my book? The view. **When**

you walk outside, you're in a world without walls, a room without a ceiling, a place so big it makes everything seem possible. So put on your sneakers, open your eyes, lift your chin, and get going. Be calmed and inspired by what you see along the way: trees swaying, clouds floating, neighbors laughing, dogs trotting. Don't waste your time debating with a spouse, friend, or yourself before you go. Yes, go for a walk. Get outside of your environment, away from your schedule, and give yourself a minute to breathe and let be. When things are looking dark from inside your windows, they might just get brighter as soon as you head out.

Fill in the easiest answer first.

Life is like a crossword puzzle in the *New York Times*. Not the easy Monday one (says the girl who can't fill in half of it), but the Sunday edition, the ultimate challenge, full of long rows of empty boxes and impossibly cryptic clues. Sometimes, your puzzle in life seems so big that you just want to rip it up and use it to line the cat box. Here's another idea: Get started on your next goal the same way you'd start one of those crosswords: Ignore the big picture for a minute, and start with the easiest answers first.

When I interviewed Will Shortz, puzzle editor for the *New York Times*, about how to complete a crossword, he said this: "Start with something you're sure of, and build from there . . .

If it's 'Charles Dickens's Blank of Two Cities,' in four letters, it has to be 'Tale.' There's *no* other word it can be, and that gives you some crossings." That works for the crossword you can carry into your life: **When the possibilities of life overwhelm you—nearly as much as a big, blank puzzle on a page—don't worry about the tough stuff that lies ahead. Just fill in the easiest answers first.**

Make one phone call, send one email, eat one healthy meal. Reach your goal one letter at a time. If you know you need to make a website, for instance, you can bury yourself under the stress of all that you need to get done—domaining, hosting, writing, planning, scanning, drawing, uploading, blogging— or you can fill in the first blank: Choose a domain name and buy it. Don't worry about what happens six steps from now, or twenty. Take the next step. And like the answer on a crossword, aim for the easiest one. If you put it down one letter and one step at a time, you'll get where you're going.

And if nothing's working? Put the puzzle aside and come back later, because sometimes with a fresh look at things, an answer will come to you that you hadn't thought of before. And if you simply don't know what first step to take, take a stab at something, *anything*. It works for puzzles and it can work for you. "Don't be afraid to guess," says Shortz. "If you're stuck in a puzzle, try something out and see if it works. Sometimes," he says, "you'll be right."

....

See plans as just blueprints.

....

Pencils may have given way to computer keys, but sometimes it helps to see our plans as always penciled in. When the picnic gets rained out, the costume you sewed needs to be two sizes bigger, or the business deal needs an overhaul to keep it from collapsing entirely, remember this: **Plans are blueprints for how you'd like something to proceed, with the understanding that life, like a client with approval rights, gets to have a last-minute say.**

So the next time your plans go south, see the change as a fussy client who absolutely loved the blueprint you've made but now thinks it would be better done, oh, completely differently. It happens. Blueprints change. The picnic is now in your living room, the costume is going to the larger kid, and that deal will be overhauled whether you'd like it to be or not.

The good news is you're much further prepped in making a new plan than you were making the first one. Think about it: When you were first planning the picnic, you didn't know who was coming, what you'd be serving, or how you'd all be feeling. Now? You know. With the business deal you have to overhaul, now you know the needs of the client, the areas you'll have to make changes, and the coffee they like to drink while they watch you do it. Most of the hard work is already done; what's left are just the finishing touches.

When I interviewed Tom Silva, general contractor of *This Old House* and *Ask This Old House*, for a story on tiling a bathroom, I had all sorts of questions about perfecting the tile work itself. But you know what he told me? "The tiling is the easy part," said Tom. "The hard part is getting it prepped. Nine times out of ten, they've used the wrong mastic, the wrong backer board, or laid on floor that wasn't flat. So get the right materials and make sure the floor you lay it on is straight and level and square. The beauty is in how you prepped the job." This is true for all our endeavors. Yes, your plans have gone sour, but you're not at square one. You've prepped the job. You have the basic blueprint. Use that to build confidence as you make the changes you need.

For my wedding years ago, I spent a month designing the perfect invitations online, at a company that promised "Invitations at Your Door in One Week!" Yet two weeks after I'd ordered them, then four, then six, they still hadn't arrived, despite assurances from the company they were "on the way." At the two-month mark, the wedding had drawn too close to wait another day, so one night, still awake at three a.m. tossing and turning with anxiety, I logged on to OvernightPrints .com and redesigned a new invite on two sides of a postcard. This time, at least, I had all the details. My floor was level and my mind was prepped, so I changed the blueprint just enough: "Our invitations never arrived," I wrote, "but we hope you still can!" I mailed off the cards in envelopes filled with the confetti of hot pink bougainvillea blooms we collected from our street, and got more positive feedback on that invite than I know I would have gotten with a traditional one.

The original invitations did arrive, by the way. Three weeks *after* we returned from our honeymoon. And they made a great fire starter for our fire pit in the backyard. So you can stray from the blueprint or, heck, just burn it entirely.

Grab the color wheel.

Last month, my husband and I were carting our luggage through the Los Angeles airport, and after passing a few plane ticket counters and feeling tense about the timing of our take-off, we rolled into the counters at Virgin America. There, the lights were low, some walls were painted magenta, the floor was lined with rug tiles, and the counters were topped with colorful vases of flowers. We felt instantly better, completely at ease. And it was a welcome reminder about the power of color to instantly change how we feel.

Years ago, for instance, I painted my former Greenwich Village living room Tiffany turquoise blue, which lightened my energy after a long day of work. I recently bought a pair of hot pink sneakers that kinda make me want to do a little jig. And my new favorite note-taking Sharpie is bright purple, which amps up an otherwise dull to-do list.

So grab the color wheel and steer yourself to a better mood. Because when we find ways to brighten our days physically, we *feel* brighter figuratively: Wear a red shirt, or a yellow dress, or carry an aqua-striped bag. Buy a pen with green ink or some sticky notes in orange. Get pillows for your couch in kelly green or sheets in tangerine. Or paint a wall in your home a shade that boosts your mood. Add color to your life on the outside and you will feel brighter inside.

Numerous studies have proven the effects color can have on our moods, actions, and how effectively we work. Changing what's around us can alter what we do.

A study by Andrew Elliot out of the University of Rochester, for example, assessed the relationship of color with creativity. Participants were presented with a booklet of anagrams to complete with their participant code printed on the corners of each page in either red, green, or black and were told to check their code in the corner of each page before solving the puzzles. In the end, the participants who were given green numbers—the color of green lights and "go"—solved nearly 30 percent more anagrams than those who were given the red—and "stop." Color "influences us at a deep biological level," Elliot told me, "in the same way it influences other primates."

As Laurel and Hardy might have said, there's gold in them thar hues. Transform your home, your workspace, your pen ink, and yourself with simple color changes. What color makes you feel happy? What color makes you feel strong? **What makes you want to wake up, get up, accomplish your goals, find moments of calm, and walk into a roomful of people with a full smile on your face, feeling your absolute best?**

It's easier to change your environment than to change your mind, right? So let your environment or your wardrobe up your mind-set in just that way. Just a few shades of difference in your everyday items can make life feel more vivid all around.

Cover your blank canvas.

My husband is an artist who paints by the name Gusto. Every day, he dips a brush in a dollop of bright paint and spreads it thoughtfully on canvas for hours, turning abstract lines into images of Marilyn Monroe, Woody Woodpecker, or a couple tango dancing in the night. My art, on the other hand, looks like an ad for *Can You Draw Better Than a Fifth Grader?* I can never seem to get the nose right, or the legs, so I fall back on stick figures to get my feelings across. But when I'm feeling melancholy, needing a dose of optimism I can't find within myself, I know what to do: Be with art. For whether you see some or make some, covering your canvas in life is an antidote to a downhearted day. That's because **art, in its creation, is a reminder of human feeling. Be it happiness, fear, dread, or delight, art makes us feel *something*. And sometimes "something" is just what we need.** When our emotions are lost or jumbled, a new perspective on how we can feel could be just what we need.

We could discuss what art really "is" for a lifetime, but whether the artist is Banksy or Gusto, a woman at the library, or you molding metal into jewelry, the creation has come from within. It is thoughts and feelings put onto canvas, paper, film—the evidence of someone *feeling* something who was driven to express it. As Stella Adler, the acting teacher whose famous pupils include Judy Garland, Marlon Brando, and

Robert De Niro, once said, "Life beats down and crushes the soul, and art reminds you that you have one."

Access art and you access yourself. You may see faces more solemn or serious or disappointed than yours, bodies more stately or bare. You may create a world more impressionistic, blurred, cubed, or bleak or capture a glimmer in an eye so different, in some small way, than what you felt before. By covering your blank canvas with something, you'll add to your day.

The next time you feel a lack in your life, put yourself in the place of art. Visit a local gallery, stroll through a sculpture garden, or scan the Google Art Project for close-ups of the classics. Or make some art yourself. Then tune into how you feel, and how special life seems.

That's what art is, after all. Unlike a cheap souvenir stamped out by a big machine, art is one person's special sweep of a brush, one of twenty limited prints, or one pattern of leaves placed just so by Andy Goldsworthy. Whether you're seeing it or making it, let art help you access a new perspective on your current situation. And yes, stick figures count.

It's more than it's not.

When you're trying to live a healthy life, it's hard not to get down on yourself. You started a diet Monday, and by Wednesday you caved for a chocolate chip cookie or two. You wanted to write ten pages or organize one corner of the attic, and you gave up to see a matinee instead. You planned to work out five days this week, and on day two, you snooze-buttoned your way through it. And then of course, you beat yourself up, declared yourself weak, and wondered what the point of trying really is.

Well, the next time you slip, do this: See that what you've already done is more than it's not, and set yourself up to do better next time.

For example, if you worked out at breakfast and ate a doughnut after dinner, it's better that you worked out and ate the doughnut than if you *hadn't* worked out and ate the doughnut; it's more than it's not. If you stopped practicing piano after learning how to play your scales, it's better that you learned to play your scales on the piano than no notes at all; it's more than it's not. **If you've done *anything* toward your goal, then you're ahead of where you were. It's more than it's not.** If you've taken one sweaty run, written one batch of pages, opened one box to organize, you're one step ahead. So pat yourself on the back and try better next time.

Your struggle with willpower is natural. As research by Roy Baumeister, Kathleen Vohs, and others has shown, our willpower depletes throughout the day. Much like a muscle, willpower can be strengthened and exhausted, depending on how it's used. Resisting a second cupcake, for instance, is like lifting a weight, and after a full day of similar decisions, you might not have it in you anymore. But there are some ways to renew yours. Studies are showing, for example, that keeping glucose levels steady helps, as does laughing and keeping your goals small; and one study out of the National University of Singapore and the University of Chicago Booth School of Business found that clenching muscles in your hands, arms, or legs at a moment of decision can give you instant willpower. (It's that embodied cognition we discussed in "Always spring for your limo": Adopt the physical posture, and the feelings will come with it.) Another way to bolster willpower comes from philosopher Chrisoula Andreou at the University of Utah, who believes we can "leverage" our self-control. Find an area of your life where you *do* have self-control and use that to leverage where you know you won't.

Let's say you eat healthy during the day, but once the sun goes down, all you want to eat are the baby Snickers bars from Halloween. Well, since you *know* this is where you lack self-control, this is where you bolster yourself so you won't need to rely 100 percent on your weakened willpower. How? Toss out those Snickers. Air-pop some popcorn and put it into sandwich bags, chop up a fruit salad, or make a hummus and precut veggies to dip in it. Now, when you're on the couch jonesing for those candy bars, you'll walk into the kitchen, low on willpower, and see only healthy snacks to gnaw on. Your willpower will barely be needed.

This works in all areas of your life: If you know you never get important work done after lunch, do the big stuff before it. If you know you'll want a cigarette after happy hour, pack some Sour Patch Kids in your bag to eat instead. If you know you won't want to go to the gym after you get home, change into your workout clothes at the office so you're not relying on your willpower to get you back out of your Snuggie.

However much good you do, congratulate yourself. *It's more than it's not.* Any small step in the right direction is better than standing still.

....

Practice self-compassion.

....

On a girls' night out, my friend Laura said she was kicking herself for not finishing a project by her self-imposed deadline. She said she was too easily distracted, called herself lazy, and said it was hopeless to think she could ever finish anything.

"Why are you being so *mean* to yourself?" one friend asked her gently. "You'd never say any of those things to *me*."

She was right. Laura would never say the cruel things to us she was saying to herself! More likely, she'd say things like, "It's okay, you've done so much already. You have a lot on your plate. It's amazing you got as far as you did." And that's the script our inner selves deserve, too. Don't be mean to yourself. Talk to yourself as kindly as you'd talk to a good friend.

But hey, we all criticize ourselves sometimes. It's natural. When I don't get the top item on my to-do list done, or I follow up a healthy dinner by polishing off a bag of chips, I'll think, *You idiot. You blew it again.* I figure my willpower didn't work, so maybe tough love will. "We think by criticizing ourselves, we're going to keep ourselves in line," says Kristin Neff, PhD, an associate professor of human development at the University of Texas at Austin and author of *Self-Compassion.*

But **self-compassion, the act of being kind to yourself, can actually motivate you more. Be your own good friend, hold your own hand, and say the right things to your own mind.** "You're still taking responsibility for your mistakes," Neff told me, "but instead of being harshly judgmental about them, you're motivating yourself to make needed changes with kindness."

It reminds me of what the character Don Draper said on an episode of *Mad Men* as he tried to spin some bad news about an advertising client: "If you don't like what's being said, change the conversation." And that's true even of a conversation you're having with yourself. If you don't like what you're telling yourself, fix it. Don't be mean to yourself another second. *You* are responsible for the words spinning around in your brain, so if you catch yourself being too negative ("I'm bound to screw this up") or accusatory ("It's my fault as usual"), then put some spin on your own story and change what's being said. Give yourself a break!

First, forgive yourself for your negative self-talk; as Neff says, "Don't beat yourself up for beating yourself up in the vain hope that it will stop you from beating yourself up!" Then imagine what you'd say to a friend going through the same situation. Hear your tone of voice, the terms of endearment. "Sweetie," you might say, "it's okay. No one could have handled what you had on your plate." Or, "You don't need to be strong about this, so go ahead and cry it out." Then turn it around on yourself and say the very same things. Or write yourself a letter from the perspective of a very compassionate friend.

However you do it, stop the self–beat down. Soften up. Be

kind. Offer yourself the same respect, warmth, forgiveness, and love that you save for the people you care about. Because, really, one of your own best friends should be you.

....

Don't take your "blah" personally.

....

I don't know about your "blah" days, but my last one went a little like this: I woke up tired and wasted forty-five minutes clicking inconsequential Internet links, and when I finally got to work, I never really seemed to get rolling. Feeling defeated, I ate an unhealthy lunch instead of an energizing one. Then I turned on the TV and watched rich people buy dream vacation homes while I lay supine on the couch in my sweats, thinking, *What in the world is the bright side of* this?

The next day, however, I was so driven by how unproductive I'd just been that I barreled through the day with a different attitude about my "blah." We need, I decided, days like that in the range of life. When we feel "blah" about what we're wearing, the weird things our hair is doing, or about how we hardly got anything productive or useful done at all, it's okay. I think the kind of day where we're not succeeding nor failing but simply not living up to our ideal is important: **A "blah" is our baseline, the steady pulse that sets the standard for our highs and lows. Without the "blah," we wouldn't even know what the "best" was**.

I like the way that Tracey Bloom, a season-seven contestant

on *Top Chef*, put it the day she was eliminated from the show. "I don't think I left because I'm a bad chef," she said. "I think I left because I had a bad day." Her bad day involved a failed pie and some burgers that went wrong, but her attitude was spot-on—and she was employing an optimistic "temporary" explanatory style that reminded her not to take her one-time failure personally. "I was not feeling it," Tracey later said. "If I could have taken a day off, I would have been fine the next day."

And that's precisely what you do on a "blah" day, too. You write it off—even if, like Tracey, you got kicked off for it. Your bad days are not a reflection of the true you forever, from this day forward. They're just off days. Don't take them to heart. The fact is, no one can be profoundly productive every day of every month of every year. We're simply not built to sustain that.

When you feel deep in the "blahs," forgive yourself. It's not you, it's life. The trees need some gray days to survive and so do we. Tomorrow, you can actively take back your life again. But today, let the lame day go and leave your "blahs" far behind.

When LIFE'S LITTLE ANNOYANCES Happen ...

Love the line.

I used to despise the lines at airports. Not being a frequent enough or rich enough traveler to earn my spot on an express lane, I'd drip with irritation and desperation. I hoped my big, heavy sigh would get us the heck checked in (it didn't), that my tapping feet would get me farther ahead (they didn't), that throwing my head back and curling my fists would send a message to the airport gods that with all the progress we've made as a human race, we didn't deserve such a backward system (well, that part's true . . . we don't). **But since I can't change the line, I decided instead to change how I feel about it. And so can you.**

I know it's not easy. I mean, come on, lines stink. A line is a lag in a smooth day, a snag in a sweater. But you know what else it could be? A little lusty moment in a well-oiled day. You could learn, if you wanted to, to love the line.

To start, answer me this: How many times have you wished there were more hours in the day, more minutes away from work, more alone time with no one other than yourself? Well, a line is your equivalent of the magic fairy who floats into your life and says, "I now grant you eight minutes to do absolutely nothing but stand here."

I know what you might be thinking: *If I had eight free minutes, I wouldn't want to spend it with strangers at the airport or the DMV or the grocery store. I'd be home with my feet up. I'd be getting a massage. I'd be sitting in a park. I'd be kissing my spouse.* But I'll wager you this: The last time you had eight free minutes, you didn't book a massage or put your feet up in a park next to your spouse. More likely, you checked your email. You picked up a magazine. You paid some bills. You read the news. You updated Facebook. Or you used your eight free minutes to help someone else.

The line is the one place you can't do the things you'd normally do on your own—and this isn't necessarily a bad thing! Stuck in a moment of staying put, you don't have access to the distractions you'd fill your day with at home or in the office. All you have is yourself and what's in your purse or pocket. So I say, use it.

The next time you're in a line, take a deep breath. You know what? Take three. Look around you at the people in line beside you. Ask yourself: What are their lives like? Where are they off to? How lucky am I to have my life today when I walk out that door? Use the time to make a mental to-do list, or an appreciative "I'm grateful for . . ." one. Focus on the hum of the people or the sun outside the window.

And when you get home, do yourself a favor and prepare yourself for your next fidgety moment with the masses. Put a magazine or a novel in your work bag. Pack thank-you notes and a pen. Pick up a sudoku puzzle book that fits in your pocket. Or charge your iPod, packed full of music or motivational speeches. "When I go to the doctor's office, I always take my knitting," my aunt JoAnne told me. "I almost feel cheated out of my quality time to knit when my name is called!"

The point is, if you're prepared to enjoy your free minutes the next time you find yourself sitting in a waiting area or snaking through a line toward airport security, you'll be the one who doesn't mind the eight minutes—or thirty-eight—it takes to get to the front of the line. You'll be the one appreciating a little life on pause and maybe even grinning because of it. Of course, then you might not get love from the frustrated customers around you, but you'll feel a little love within yourself.

Love the line and you might just start to look forward to it.

Thank the lemons.

When my sister, Liz, was looking for a new house to rent with a friend, her wish list looked like many of ours: a clean interior, a cute yard space, and a cozy feel. But on the first day of her search, she saw two houses with no yards, few windows, and unusual layouts. The homes may have been right for someone, but they weren't her cup of tea.

It took a few more appointments before she saw some more right ones for her, and only then did she realize how glad she was to have seen the wrong ones. For when she found her perfect home, how else would she have been able to appreciate it without having the others to compare them to? **It's as simple as this: You'll never be able to appreciate the sweet stuff if you haven't had some lemons.**

This is true of everything in life. You won't know a great job if you've never worked a crappy one. You can't savor a nice hotel if you've never stayed in a dirty one. You'll never appreciate your health unless you or someone you love has lost it. And how could you value a wonderful, stomach-swirling date if you've never had some clunkers?

Like my sister's house hunt, look at your low moments in life as setting a gauge for the highs. Being in a job that beats you down can teach you that you deserve to be working for one where you soar. Kissing someone who doesn't summon an iota of chemistry within you can remind you that, yeah, you *want* the butterflies. And running into bitter lemons on a search for the perfect four-door car or full-time nanny is the only way to recognize success when you see it.

After Liz signed the lease on the house she loved, she was able to look back on those other houses with gratitude. That's because, in time, the things that are *so* not right for us become our most revelatory or most touching or funniest experiences. Thank the lemons. As sour as they are, they'll help you appreciate the true sweetness of life.

Re-appreciate the redo.

My friend Dreux was slogging through an eight-hour drive when he got off the interstate for some coffee. Unfortunately, he got back on headed the wrong way and didn't realize it until he'd driven a straight hour in the wrong direction.

Ouch, right? But redos like this happen all the time. You just vacuumed the rug when someone spills chips on it. You just composed a thoughtful email or an entire term paper before your computer went down. Or, like the recent morning Gus and I spent shopping for the barbecue we were hosting, we don't realize until our guests have arrived that we forgot the most important item at the store: the charcoal. None of us want to do something we *just* did all over again. So how do we handle it?

You take three deep breaths, lift your chin, and say this: "I'm going to get something *else* out of it this time." Because

maybe this redo is the universe saying you missed something the first time. Maybe this time, you can squeeze more out of it. If you choose to get something else out of it the second time around, it will no longer be wasted time. With ingenuity and a new attitude, it can be a new experience entirely.

If you have to drive back to the market for some milk, take the road past that old house you've always loved or tune to a symphony or an eighties song you sing all the way to the parking lot. Maybe you call a funny friend and say, "I only have four minutes, but I'm having the most frustrating day and I really just wanted to hear your voice." Or you decide that on this trip, you'll be more giving than ever: You'll stop for jaywalking pedestrians, let people cut in front of you, and ask the cashier how his day is going.

The second time you vacuum, turn on some samba music and dance with it. The second time you put the deleted names back into your phone, do it outside on your front porch in the sun. The second time you write an email, make it even better, cleaner, and sharper than the first. There are ways to make the second time around different, and possibly even—in a stretch, perhaps—better.

However you can do it, re-appreciate the redo. Find what it is the universe thinks you missed the first time around. Sure, it may take some stomping, growling, and yelling before you get started, but when your breathing is back to normal, inhale slowly and say to yourself, "I'm going to get something else out of it this time." The second time can be a better time if you take the opportunity to find out how.

....

At least you're not . . .

....

Soon after attorney Ian Graham was hired at Latham and Watkins, he was placed on a pro bono case representing Mario Rocha, who at sixteen was wrongfully accused of shooting a teen outside of a party and was serving two life sentences for a crime he didn't commit.

"The first time I met Mario in prison," Ian told me, "I was a second-year lawyer with no social life because I was pounded with work. Then I visited Mario in Calapatria State Prison in the desert near the California/Mexico border. It was a total epiphany for me," Ian said. "Here was a guy about my age and as intelligent if not more so than I was, and because he was in the wrong place at the wrong time, he was in prison for a crime he didn't commit, and handling it with grace and a belief that things would work out for him."

By the time Ian got in his nice car to drive to his nice house in Santa Monica, he thought, *You gotta be kidding me that I'm worrying about working so hard and how I don't have the right furniture in my place while he's in prison for ten years for something he didn't do.* It was the fast track to gratitude.

Ian's epiphany is an example of how one single shift in your perspective can help you appreciate what you have. At least you have your health, or your safety, or your legs, or your life. **When you're in a bad place or a bad mood, find something you're glad hasn't happened that could have been worse. "At least I'm not . . ." makes all the difference.**

Did you just get a flat tire? At least you're not on the highway. If you are on the highway? At least you're not in a snowstorm, fifty miles outside of any town. And if you *do* get a flat tire in a snowstorm fifty miles outside of any town, at least your tire didn't blow out, spin you into a barrier, and pin you behind the wheel. There is always a worse place to be, and by reminding yourself how lucky you are, your perception will change. As my sister-in-law, Mariana, said one day as we crawled through traffic past an accident on a Florida highway, "All I can say is, at least we're not the ones in the accident *causing* the traffic." For whether your glass is only half full or half empty, at least it has something in it at all.

I even use an "At least I'm not . . ." when I'm trying to fall asleep on a tossy-turny night, stressing about why I'm not drifting into dreamland. Yes, I've tried picturing myself on a calm beach by a trickling stream, but that doesn't work for me. What does? Appreciating where I'm *not*. As I lay there, I'll think, *At least I'm not on a subway platform in high heels waiting twenty minutes for a train.* Or, *At least I'm not in an uncomfortable airport chair waiting for my flight to be rebooked.* Essentially, *At least I'm not in some place where all I'd wish is that my head was resting on a soft pillow under a fluffy duvet like it is right now.*

Mario's story has a happy ending, by the way. As Graham explains in his book *Unbillable Hours*, Mario's charges were vacated in 2005; he was finally freed and went on to attend George Washington University on a full scholarship. And as stressful as any class there might have gotten for him, I can only imagine Mario was grateful to be in a classroom at all. Think about this when you're in a bad situation. Really, it truly *could* be worse. At least, right now, it's not.

Recognize your new route is better.

My friend Laurie wanted to see a band called the Black Keys in Los Angeles and assumed her sister would get her a ticket. Well, all "you know what happens when you assume" jokes aside, Laurie ended up on a long search for tickets by herself on Craigslist. And she not only found one, but she made a great friend out of it.

"I met the guy at Starbucks to pick it up, and when he walked up, I thought he was adorable," says Laurie. "We sat for thirty minutes chatting about music before I bought his ticket and went to the show. He texted me the next day to see if I had fun, and we got to talking so much that I invited him to go to a Spoon show with me. We've been great friends ever since!" Her route to that concert was a circuitous one and she learned something that day we could all benefit from: **Sometimes the**

roundabout route life sends you on is better than the straight path you'd planned.

And this is the case in so many ways when you don't get what you ordered in life. Your pizza comes with pepperoni instead of peppers, the boots you ordered look different than they did on the website, and the life you thought you were going to live is no longer in the cards. These are glitches in the factory conveyer belt of life. But just because the outcome wasn't the one you "ordered" doesn't mean it will be grim. It's entirely possible the new route you've been sent down will be even better than the first.

My friend Kerry can attest to this. Six years into her career in television ad sales, she got a fab new corporate job headed to the big-time; but a few months in, she started getting heart palpitations and vertigo, and felt so fatigued she couldn't drive herself home. She had CAT scans and MRIs and wore a heart monitor to pinpoint the cause, but things only got worse as Kerry developed cysts on her wrists that required her to wear splints and made it impossible to type. "I'd been so motivated to kick ass at my new job and prove myself," Kerry told me, "and there I was, barely able to make it through a workday." Finally, after a visit to an allergist, she got her diagnosis: A mold from the office was making her ill. Armed with her answer, Kerry steered hard to stay on course: She switched offices, got a dehumidifier, took allergy medicine, and went for treatment on her wrists. But she had to face the fact that this was no way to work—which is when she wondered if her heart was really in advertising at all.

Kerry had gone to school for fashion marketing and was always sketching ideas for swimsuits. And though she'd never had formal training in fashion design itself, she left her office one day and bought some fabrics, then sewed some samples and sent them to the annual swim show in Miami. Weeks later, to the hum of her humidifier in the office, she got a call from the fashion bible *Women's Wear Daily* wanting to interview her for a story. That was all the encouragement she needed. Kerry quit her advertising job, got her health back, and kept sewing. When the article came out, Saks Fifth Avenue called her in for a meeting; and at the swim show in Miami, she got her first order from the hip boutique Kitson. Six years later, Kerry Cushman's Kushcush suits have been worn by Kim Kardashian and featured in *Sports Illustrated*, and her career is even better than she'd dreamed.

"When I look back on it now, this was always the path I was supposed to be on," says Kerry. "It just took a weird and slightly traumatic experience to get here. It was like my body was telling me that *wasn't* what I was supposed to be doing—and giving me the chance to do what I'd always wanted: fashion." What seemed like a roadblock for Kerry was actually a redirect to a better path. She just had to let go of the wheel and let life steer her in the right direction.

When life sends you on a different route, it's natural to wish things had happened as you planned. But maybe the route you're on now is even better. Maybe the scenery is prettier on a side road, or you'll learn things you couldn't have on the busy highway. Maybe who you're meeting and what you're experiencing will ultimately bring you closer to true happiness. So turn off that nagging GPS voice telling you to make a U-turn and, like Laurie and Kerry, see the riches your roundabout route gives you, too.

Ask, where *doesn't* it hurt?

You know that old joke: A guy walks into a doctor's office and says, "My arm hurts when I move it like this."

"Well then," says the doctor, "don't move it like that."

It's humorously bad advice, but it does offer us some insight on dealing with small temporary pain in our lives. Sometimes, the more you focus on the pain you're feeling or about to feel, the more you notice it. So here's what I might also tell that guy in the doctor's office: Think about your *other* arm. **When you're feeling some temporary pain in one area of your body, be grateful for a part of your body that isn't feeling it. Where *doesn't* it hurt?**

I use this all the time. When my dental hygienist is scraping my top teeth so much that my upper gums are starting to throb, I think about how good my lower gums feel. When the cloth from a bikini wax is about to be ripped from my right side, I think about how pain-free I am on my left. When I'm getting acupuncture needles inserted in my leg, I focus on my hand. And when a nurse is taking blood from my left arm, I look at the same untouched spot on my right.

The way I see it, it's like trying to tune into the senses of smell and taste at the same exact time; you can't. (Seriously, try it, you really can't!) Yes, they work in unison. But by focusing on your taste, you lose the ability to tune into your smell and vice versa. With pain, we can make this choice subjectively: By focusing on your right foot, you cannot give as much credence to your left, and by focusing on the hand that isn't being pricked with a needle, you simply can't give your full attention to the one that is. Perhaps, then, some of the small pain we feel is relative to the feelings we have about it.

"We convert pain into suffering in the mind," writes Howard C. Cutler, MD, coauthor with the Dalai Lama, in *The Art of Happiness*. "There is a difference," he writes, "between physical pain, which is a physiological process, and suffering, which is our mental and emotional response to the pain. So the question arises: Can finding an underlying purpose and meaning behind our pain modify our attitude about it? And can a change in attitude lessen the degree to which we suffer when we are physically injured?" For those pokes and plucks and scrapes and bruises, can changing how we think affect how it feels? Can thinking about the arm that doesn't hurt help the suffering of the one that does? I think so. And I think it can also work with what taxes us emotionally.

If you're hitting a rough patch in the relationship area of your life, maybe your work or social life *doesn't* hurt. If your car battery died and you need a new starter—and, actually, those tires are ready for a change—maybe your home hasn't given you headaches or you feel healthy while everyone else is fighting the flu. Relieve yourself of some suffering by focusing on the place you're not feeling it. Where doesn't it hurt?

Like the guy in the doctor's office, you may never be so grateful for an arm—or a heartbreak—that *doesn't* hurt when you move it like that.

Create calm in your storm.

I'd just climbed into a taxi when I got an exasperating email and found myself cursing like a sailor in the backseat for a minute.

"I'm so sorry," I said. "My normal cursing-to-regular-words ratio in life is only about one percent, but in your cab, it's been about twenty."

"At *least*!" the driver replied.

I laughed and toned it back down to zero, but two things occurred to me. One, a study I'd read about that found profanity eases your pain. (Seriously, a study by Richard Stephens at Keele University published in *NeuroReport* in 2009 determined that participants who repeated a curse word as frequently and as loudly as they wanted while keeping their hands in buckets of ice-cold water were able to endure it 40 percent longer and reported feeling less pain than those allowed to utter neutral words about, say, a table.) But while we might feel better for a minute, yelling at a phone, screaming at cars in traffic, or kicking a dining chair during a fight doesn't help us move forward. So once you get your NC-17 rant out of your system, seek the calm in your storm. Calm yourself *mentally* by calming yourself *physically*. Here's what I mean.

When you're emotionally fed up, your sympathetic nervous system jumps to attention in "fight-or-flight" mode: Your muscles tighten, your heart races, your breathing increases, and adrenaline rushes through your body, preparing you to battle your stressful situation. So, **if you'd rather feel calm in the storm, run the course in reverse: Physiologically change how your body *feels* so you emotionally react more calmly.** This way, you're activating your parasympathetic nervous system, which relaxes your muscles, slows your breathing, and calms you down.

If you physiologically behave as a calm and relaxed person, you will bring on that emotional state; you'll trick your body into believing the *un-hype*. So when you're about to lose it—in traffic, during an argument, at work, or on the phone—here are some ways to gain composure and calm:

- Take three long, slow, and very deep breaths that fully contract your diaphragm.

- Relax your face—especially your forehead and jaw, where we hold a lot of our tension. Use one free hand to rub your forehead and jaw into relaxation.

- Generate a big smile for fifteen seconds that pulls at the zygomaticus and orbicularis oculi muscles on either side of your eyes—the ones that create your crow's-feet—and you'll unconsciously send signals to your emotional brain that you're feeling happier.

- Stretch your arm up over your head or across your body like a good old-fashioned Jane Fonda workout warm-up.

- Play calming music. Los Angeles composer Ken Elkinson created *Music for Commuting*, a six-CD set of ambient music for his own daily commutes. "I'm an angry driver," Ken admits. "I'm the one screaming at people to put on their signals, so I wanted something to relax me while I drove." Use what works for you.

- Call a friend or family member who makes you laugh.

- Force a yawn. A 2008 study of yawning parakeets published in *Animal Behaviour* found yawning is a way to cool down a heated brain, the way you would a hot computer. Cooler heads prevail, right? Yawn your way there.

In addition to the things you can do physically to create a calm in your storm, you can also alter your environment. When I have a big deadline for work, for instance, and I worry I'll never get it done, I look at my body language. Yep, there I am, pacing the house, biting my nails, frantically scrubbing dishes to redirect my stress. So I create a calming space—the environment version of deep breathing. I light a fig-scented candle, play some old Dinah Washington, slip on a fuzzy cashmere sweater and comfy socks, and pour myself a hot cup of tea. By creating calm around me, I silence the storm with an atmosphere around my desk that sings like an old lullaby, *You are so calm and relaxed it's not even funny.*

So whether you're fuming at a traffic jam, riled up in your relationship, or just plain stressed to the max, counteract your frustration by reversing the route that got you there. Calm your body and your environment, and you will calm your mind.

See life like a seesaw.

As Newton's third law of motion says, for every action, there is an equal and opposite reaction. In physics, energy doesn't disappear, it is transferred. Well, we can look at life the same way. Where there's a loss, there's a benefit. It's like a seesaw really: When one side of life feels weighed down, there may be another side lifting up. The rain that's washing out your picnic is watering the plants, after all, and another day's blazing hot weather is at least making it warm enough to swim. Somewhere, there is a benefit; somehow, there is gain.

Say, for example, you drop an envelope containing $100 in cash. Ouch, I know. But whether that money was going for a phone bill or a much-needed treat, your loss is now on life's seesaw where the next ride up is going to someone else: Where you lost that envelope, someone else found it. Where you are hanging your head low with disappointment, someone is calling Mom with untold delight. Yes, maybe some selfish jerk found the money, but maybe someone just like *you* found it—someone just like you reached down to get their soda from a sticky movie theater floor and found themselves the beneficiary of your bad day. Your loss has been their gain. And as the world's karma supply shifts again in the future, the reverse will be true. Someday, that gain will be yours. It's the seesaw of life wherever you are.

When the person you love chooses someone else, it's the seesaw of love: The loss you're feeling now is only opening you up for the gain of a future partner who loves you to absolute pieces. You'll *both* be better off for the love you'll get to have.

And when you're stuck at a stoplight watching cars flow through the green, it's the seesaw of traffic patterns: Today is their lucky day; today it's their turn. Next week, you'll be flying through the intersection, driving the open highway east while the westbound traffic sits at a standstill.

Somewhere, somehow, in every moment in life, where there is emptiness in one place, there is fullness in another. We're one seesaw, sharing our energy with one another, taking turns in losses and getting our chance at the gains. Someday, you'll find what someone else has left behind. Be it money or a book, a lost puppy or a rejected lover; be it a job, a spot in a school program, or first place in a 5K, someday you'll gain. Someday *you'll* be the beneficiary of someone else's loss. So now, try to graciously give the benefits to someone else.

We each get our time on the top of the seesaw sometime. Just endure this down until your next ride up.

....

High-five your failures.

....

My family still talks about "The Great Wine Experiment." It was around 1978 when my dad brainstormed a way to make the Cabernet he uncorked on day one taste just as good two weeks later. "I wondered if I put nitrogen into the wine bottle to purge the oxygen, if it would prevent oxidation," my dad said.

So he bought a cylinder of nitrogen to test his theory. They didn't have a regulator in stock, the device placed over the nitrogen valve that would reduce the 1,800 psi (pounds per square inch) pressure to, say, 10 psi. He figured he'd adjust the pressure himself.

That night, he opened a bottle of wine and replaced the cork with a contraption that attached one piece of rubber tubing to the nitrogen tank, and rested the other in the wineglass. We all watched, giddy with anticipation.

What was supposed to happen: As he gently cracked the valve open on the nitrogen bottle, the nitrogen was supposed to flow into the wine bottle, and push the wine up the glass tube and through the rubber tubing *into* the glass, which would have worked beautifully at ten psi.

What actually happened: As he tried to crack the valve open the *slightest* bit so the nitrogen would gently push the wine into the glass, the valve stuck. So he turned a bit harder. At which point something closer to 1,800 psi of nitrogen— equivalent to the pressure of a power washer you'd use to clean your outdoor deck and siding—shot into the wine bottle. "There was so much force," my dad says, "that the rubber tube jumped out of the wineglass and started wildly waving around, spraying wine all over the kitchen ceiling, walls, and cabinets. I shut it off as quickly as I could, but those few seconds had already made their mark." It was an epic failure that led to hours of cleanup. (We *still* find specks of wine on the cabinets.) But it also led to a rejigging of the device that's worked perfectly for three decades and years of laughs.

From now on, think of your failures as reasons to celebrate. Like the punch holes you earn on your way to a free ride, your failures are worth a big high five.

Mistakes like that are how we learn. And whether at work, in art, in love, or in creativity, we *have* to make our own. Look at your next undertaking as an experiment, too. For if you blow it at first, you'll learn more for the next time. Failure can be fun when you see it from the right angle. And whether you're cleaning up wine or healing your ego, high-five yourself for being one punch hole closer to getting it right.

Rally in the rain delay!

Ah, the baseball game. The smell of fresh-cut grass and stadium food. The sound of the "beer here" guy making his rounds. The feeling of spring in the air and . . . wait, is that a raindrop?

Is that two? For then, as the drizzle turns to a downpour, you also get a taste for what else an outdoor sport has to offer: the rain delay. It's Mother Nature's call whether she'll sprinkle the field for ten minutes or two hours, but how you spend the time is all up to you.

What do you do during the rain delay? Do you sit in your seat and complain with your arms crossed for an hour while your sneakers puddle with water? No. You rally. You go inside and pay $11 for a hot dog that's so long you need two hands (and two buns, really) to eat it. You strike up a conversation with your fellow fans. You post what you're up to online or call a friend or watch the news on the monitors inside while you wait out the holdup. Well, learn from yourself. **Like a rain delay in life, the next time you're stuck in traffic, waiting for a late bus, or praying for the cable to come back on, find a way to rally to pass the time.** Basically, resign yourself to the suckiness and focus on something else. Because if all you do is focus on the rain in your way, you'll work yourself into a grumbling, stressed-out mess. Distract yourself right out of it instead.

When Gus and I were driving to host an art event at his loft downtown, we ran into a standstill on the highway, traffic snarled and crawling two miles to the next exit. We knew right away that our thirty-minute drive would take an hour and a half. So we called our friend Johnny White to watch the fort, then did what comes naturally: We sulked. We seethed. And we complained about the cars around us ("Uh, hello, does merge mean *nothing* to you?") and the mess we were in ("Man, we are screwed. We are *so* screwed."). But with nothing to do but wait for the rain delay of the traffic to abate, we realized our mind-set was only making us feel worse. So, we rallied.

"Okay," Gus said, "what do we do?"

We played Kiss, Marry, Kill with characters from our favorite TV shows; then, realizing how weird it is to play a game about who you'll kiss and marry with someone you're married *to*, we moved on to Twenty Questions; then, a few rounds of Radio Roulette to see who could be first to guess the songs as we scanned through the stations. I won't say we had so much fun we didn't notice the traffic, but the ride only felt half as long. That's the thing with a rain delay: If you resign yourself to the suckiness and distract yourself, you simply won't be able to get as riled up. Look around. See what can calm you down. This is what Hangman and Tic-Tac-Toe and iPod mixes of songs you know by heart were made for.

When my guy friends had to wait an hour for a table at a popular sushi place, they set up a paperclip hockey game on the sidewalk and were laughing so hard before dinner that they almost missed their name being called. And when my girl-friend missed her afternoon train connection to the Hamptons and had to wait three hours for the next one in Queens, she walked a few blocks to a pub, hoisted herself onto a barstool, and declared it beer o'clock.

Sometimes, life will rain on your parade, throw detours on the highway, knock out your Internet, and strand you on the side of the road with an overheated engine until AAA comes to your aid. What happens next is up to you: You can turn it into an excuse to complain or consider it a challenge on how to pass the time. Rally through the rain delay. You never know, you might have an okay time before the first pitch is even thrown.

Put a bow on it for your future self.

Years ago, my sister flew to Mexico for some work as a massage therapist. Seeing the large group of people she'd be working with who'd known each other for years, Liz felt like the new kid in high school. And because she was working in near isolation in a small office, she found it hard to get to know people and a little loneliness started setting in. Two weeks later, she had one *really* bad day. During a walk alone along the ocean, she was chased by a wild dog and bitten on the leg.

Liz rushed back to the hotel and got a ride to the hospital for a tetanus shot. And although she was gripped with pain and fear that day, something positive slowly began to unravel: One by one, people in the group started popping into her office, reaching out, and introducing themselves.

"I heard about the bite," people would say. "Are you okay?"

By the end of the week, in fact, she'd met everyone she'd be working with and finally felt at ease. Admittedly, says Liz, "I wasn't able to recognize the benefits of that dog bite until years later, but it helps me to this day." How? "I've thought since," she says, 'why did it take a *dog bite* for me to get to know people?' Now, on a job, I'll introduce myself as soon as I can so I feel more comfortable right off the bat."

What happened in my sister's past—a wild dog attack and a tetanus shot in another country—has helped her in her future. And we have the ability to see our bad luck the same way. You know the last tricky thing that happened to you? Well, your future self called and wants to tell you something: "Thank you."

Your experiences today are not for naught. As grueling or tiring or defeating as something might feel today, it is providing invaluable riches for your future self. So wrap it up and put a big bow on it to hand it to your future you. **Because if you can't see a benefit in your present, then you're at least giving a present to your future.**

Say you went through a heart-shattering breakup. As you grieve, take comfort in knowing your future self thanks you—for you are, with every tear, becoming a more feeling and heartful person, more empathetic than you've ever been before. Will your future self also be more wary about opening your heart so you don't get hurt again? Absolutely. But there are gains. For your future self, cuddled up comfortably with the partner of your dreams, is sorry you're so sad about it, but grateful beyond measure that things didn't work out.

Everything you do today—successful or flailing—is a gift

to your future self. Getting lost on the way to the doctor today saves your future self from getting lost when it could be worse. Flubbing an interview today teaches your future self to prepare better next time so you'll soar when it's a job you'll want more. Running out of gas today reminds your future self to keep that tank a quarter full next time.

Every single thing you see, do, and maybe slip up on, is a lesson, an experience, and a gift to the future you. So get a bag of bows and start wrapping.

Save the laugh for later.

Years ago, my mom had a really bad day with some chocolate cream pies.

She and my father were invited to dinner at their friend's house, and my mom offered to bring a pie, so she made a piecrust from scratch, filled it with fluffy chocolate, topped it with freshly made whipped cream, and rested it on the lid of the outdoor barbecue to cool.

An hour before it was time to go, she opened the back door to grab the pie and stopped in shock: There, on the barbecue grill, was a squirrel *eating* the pie—cream, chocolate, crust, the works. She was crushed and wanted to crumble, but she'd promised a pie and was going to deliver.

So she made a new piecrust, mixed some new chocolate,

whipped some more cream, and created the pie all over again. With two minutes to spare, my mom walked to the car to wait for my dad. Then, remembering something else she wanted to bring, she placed the brand-new pie on the hood of the car and raced back indoors.

That's when my dad came outside, thought he saw a drip under the car, and without hesitation popped opened the hood to investigate.

"Dink!" went the sound in the driveway. *Gasp!* went my mom in the hall.

Then she raced out to see her fear realized: There was the pie tin, facedown in a halo of whipped cream on the blacktop.

This was not—I repeat, not—funny at the time. It got a notch funnier when my parents showed up to dinner late with a frozen pie they picked up along the way and it's funnier every year since.

Sometimes, things happen that are so trying, so maddening, so exasperating or embarrassing that you're not laughing about it now and you're sure you never will. But some of those times, it *is* going to be funny later, and just knowing this can help ease the pain. How will you know?

Well, you'll know because you're oddly injured (say, you walk into a sliding glass door) or you're hugely embarrassed (your zipper is down or your skirt flies up) or you're driven to cry over a circumstance that doesn't usually make adults cry (you spill milk, your heel snaps off, or you find yourself jumping up and down on an aluminum pie plate in the middle of a driveway). Chances are, when you're starting to whimper or looking to hide, it probably *will* be funny later.

Just hold on to the memory and pull it out when you're ready. Because if my mom's experience with those chocolate cream pies is any indication, what a good laugh it will be.

When Your CAREER
Isn't Going Your Way . . .

Rest for a minute . . . maybe two.

Boy, we get tired in life, don't we? Tired of researching. Tired of dating. Tired of working out. Tired of negotiating our way through red tape. And when you're that tired, what do you need? Rest. The problem is, we often don't give it to ourselves.

If I rest, you think, *how will I sign a new client? How will I sell the car? How will I find love?* I'm here to tell you that the only way to be our best and get the best is by giving ourselves a chance to rest. Let yourself off the hook.

If you're tired of planning, go rogue. If you're tired of dressing up, go natural. If you're tired of meeting new people, grab dinner with old friends. And if you're tired of hoping for the best, give yourself a break and *rest.*

Rest is not only a good idea, it's a survival necessity. Think about it: One-third of every day is spent sleeping; in a twenty-four-hour period, our bodies are meant to rest for eight of them. When you're sleeping, the organs revive, the brain consolidates and takes a vacation, and the body goes through a cycle of total rejuvenation so you can start fresh in the morning. In the Old Testament story of Genesis, God created light, sky, water, stars, meat, and popcorn in the first six days, and on the seventh day he rested—yep, even the big guy needed a nap.

Allow yourself the same with your life. **If you're feeling tapped out, over it, or tired of reaching for your goal in the first place, it's high time to rest—either in mind or body.** Rest your mind by engaging in other activities: Step away from the computer, slow down your pace, and do a 180 from the task that's tiring you out. Take a quiet stroll outside, play a game of Frisbee, read a book, grab coffee with a friend, go to a movie, or take your dog for an extra long walk. And take a literal rest, too. Find a way to get eight or more hours of sleep one night or to sneak in rejuvenating nap on a weekend afternoon. Because sleep is necessary for memory consolidation, while you may want to cram for a speech long into the night, the best thing you can do for your brain is to get some z's or think about something else.

When my friend Todd, for instance, was preparing to tell a story about growing up gay in Alabama in front of seven hundred people for the Moth, one of New York City's famous storytelling events, he was told not to practice the day of the performance. Only two people had ever frozen up at the microphone at the Moth, he was told, and both had practiced their stories that very same day. So Todd gave it a rest, then took his place onstage and let his story flow from his memory like moonshine.

Stepping away from your task may seem to potentially hinder your progress, but sometimes taking a break from the route will help you find a *better* way to get there. There was, for example, a study done at Middlesex University in London that found that participants who engaged in twenty-five minutes of exercise boosted scores on creativity tests more than participants who watched a task-related video. It's evidence of what refueling the mind can do: The minute you step back from the frontlines, you can see your goal from an entirely different angle.

Look at rest as the Saturday and Sunday to your workweek, and give your task its own personal weekend. Rest to revive and rejuvenate your mind and body so you'll be raring to go all over again.

Find your sweet spot.

Tennis players, baseball stars, and golfers know a lot about the sweet spot. Because on every tennis racquet, baseball bat, and golf club, there is a small spot from which, essentially, the maximum amount of energy is returned to the ball instead of into vibrations back through the racquet, bat, or club. The hitter will feel they've sent the ball soaring with the perfect dose of power and strength—much different from the thud I'm used to when I play paddle tennis and a hit leaves my hand tingling. And life is full of powerful pockets like this, too. There's a sweet spot to everything. The key is to find yours.

Me, I used to be a night owl. And when it came to work, I liked writing by candlelight long after dark. But one morning, waking early to meet a deadline, I found myself working faster and more efficiently than ever. I've since learned that seven to ten a.m. is my sweet spot of productivity, when it feels like I'm hitting the ball solid and far, so I slide my biggest projects into that slot, and work my way down from there.

If we don't know our sweet spots, we do have help. Physiologically, our circadian rhythms regulate our body temperature, energy, and sleep at regular cycles throughout the day, directing us to some sweet spots by dictating the best times for certain activities. According to the American Council on Exercise, for example, the best time to work out is when our body temperature is at its highest in the afternoon; this is when muscles are more flexible and our strength is at its peak. That said, we also have completely different jobs, schedules, families, and sleep cycles. So the key is to find *your* unique sweet spots and aim to hit them every time. **The more often we're hitting our sweet spots in work, relationships, learning, and fun, the happier we allow ourselves to be.**

Find your own sweet spot in productivity: What one hour

of every day does work flow easily and the distractions are minimal? Just add one to two hours on either end and you've got yourself a productive window to get things done.

In love or dating, when are you most positive and affectionate? If you and your partner feel happiest when you're taking a walk or riding bikes together, use that sweet spot if you have to talk about something serious. And when it comes to sex, find your ideal timing there, too. I know very few people who say their sweet spot for sex lies in the fifteen minutes they're climbing into bed, eyes half-mast and energy zilch. Maybe your sweet spot is before dinner instead of after it or on weekend afternoons.

Find your sweet spot of confidence, of physical strength, of willpower, of creativity. Harness the power of your sweet spots and you can hit your whole life out of the park.

Lower your standards. Sort of.

Two years ago, I picked up a gorgeously ratty Louis XV armchair at a thrift shop in town that just needed some refinishing and new upholstery to shine like new. And instead of paying a professional to do the job, I decided to take my own untrained stab at it for fun. Then a friend reminded me that there are classes for these things, and Internet videos, and that in no time, I could get the right tools and become an expert at it.

"Because if it's worth doing," he reminded me, "it's worth doing right."

So I put down my unsharpened shears and began to research upholstery techniques and what professional tools I needed, and upcoming classes I could take in the area. Well, you should see that chair now. It looks . . . exactly the same. Except on the days it's buried under a stack of clean laundry. The problem was, I got so caught up in wanting to do my upholstery project perfectly, I didn't start the project at all—when the truth is that anything I did to that chair would have been an improvement! Now, every time I place some folded towels on it, that chair is a reminder that maybe a little is better than nothing. Maybe an imperfect effort is better than no effort at all. **Am I suggesting you lower your standards? Well, yeah, I kind of am. At least I'm saying lower your standards for *starting*.** Look at your next big goal and decide to do less than you think you can achieve. Once you get started, you may find you can't help but produce something better. But either way, a started something is better than nothing at all.

In the book *Art & Fear*, authors David Bayles and Ted Orland tell the story of a ceramics teacher who conducted an experiment by dividing his class into two groups. Students on one side of the studio would be graded only on the quantity of work they produced—so that fifty pounds of pots weighed on the teacher's scale would earn an A, forty would earn a B, and so on. Students on the other side would be graded on the quality of one perfect pot at the end of the semester.

"Well," write the authors, "come grading time and a curious

fact emerged: The works of highest quality were all produced by the group being graded by quantity. It seems that while the 'quantity' group was busily churning out piles of work—and learning from their mistakes—the 'quality' group had sat theorizing about perfection, and in the end had little more to show for their efforts than grandiose theories and a pile of dead clay." The same is true in work, in dreams, in love. Don't let inexperience or fear you might do it wrong stall you. Lower your standards for starting and just get *doing*.

Sure, your first draft of your Great American Novel may not be great, but you're better off churning out a bunch of "eh" pages like piles of pottery than staring at a blank screen perfecting an opening line. And, sure, your new living room might not be perfectly planned, but the only way to know what will work in the room is to grab the couch and start pulling. And that first date might be awkward, but arranging it gives you a reason to put on a clean shirt or some lip gloss, and to dive into different experiences with new people—where you might just be pleasantly surprised.

Like the lottery, you gotta be in it to win it. You won't get any closer to perfect if you don't start. Great only happens after you've done a rough draft, or started upholstering a wonky chair, or dated some duds so you know what you're really looking for in a partner. Forget perfect on day one and lower your standards for diving in. Good things come from getting started.

Don't aim for a winner every time.

In Andre Agassi's autobiography *Open*, he recounts what his future tennis coach Brad Gilbert once said of his game. "You always try to be perfect," Gilbert told him, "and you always fall short, and it f—s with your head. Your confidence is shot, and perfectionism is the reason. You try to hit a winner on every ball, when just being steady, consistent, meat and potatoes, would be enough to win ninety percent of the time."

He's right. Would you rather have a one-hit wonder of a life, or a consistent one making music for decades? "There's about five times a year you wake up perfect," Gilbert went on with Agassi, "when you can't lose to anybody, but it's not those five times a year that make a tennis player. Or a human being, for that matter. It's the other times."

Instead of aiming for perfection every second, let go a little. Sure, you want the perfect home, relationship, career, and kids. But striving for perfect in all areas of your life can not only drive you nuts, it can hinder your happiness. Because if you can't be satisfied with a really great meal or a wonderful view or a good-quality job on your part, you'll never reach a place of satisfaction in life enough to sit back, smile, and enjoy it! And you'll never, believe it or not, succeed. "The perfectionist is never satisfied," writes Tal Ben-Shahar, PhD, in his book *Being Happy*. "She consistently sets goals and standards that are for all intents and purposes impossible to meet, thereby from the outset *rejecting the possibility of success*. No matter what she achieves . . . she can never take any pleasure in her accomplishments. No matter what she has . . . it is never good enough for her."

So your paint job isn't perfect and your partner doesn't like camping the way you do. Don't hold off on happiness until your life is absolutely, ideally picture-perfect, because you'll never, ever be happy if you do.

Does perfect happen? Sure it does. The first time I tried the crab claws in wine sauce at Mandina's in New Orleans, I knew I'd found perfect, topped with bread crumbs and a touch of butter. And when I say "touch" I mean "pound." But the dish stands out because true perfection only pops up every once in a while. Instead of making yourself nuts aiming for perfect every time, put out a darn great version of you. Don't worry about the dust bunnies under the couch, the wrinkle in your shirt, the cornbread you didn't make from scratch, the PowerPoint presentation you could have made better if you gave it more time. No one else expects or needs those things to be perfect to love you. So stop measuring how much you love yourself by how close to perfect you think you've become.

You know what perfection really is? Finding happiness in the floor models of life: "As is." Like Agassi, you don't have to hit a winner every time. Sometimes, sitting back and enjoying your magnificent life, full of imperfections and almost theres, is what winning is really all about.

....

What's your why?

....

Every time I start a new workout plan, I always hit a rough spot pretty early. Like, say, at minute nine on day one of a thirty-day plan. *This is hard,* I'll think. *Why am I doing this again?*

When you find yourself asking the same thing about your health, dare yourself to answer. Because focusing on the why can be enough to plow through the how. And like a four-year-old who never gives up, keep asking, "Why? But why? But *why*?"

"Self," you might say, "why am I working out and eating healthy again?"

"So you'll lose weight."

"Why do I want to lose weight?"

"So you'll feel better about yourself."

"Why will I feel better about myself?"

"Because you'll prove to yourself you can stick to a goal. Because your jeans will fit better and you'll feel confident wearing them. Because your increased energy will allow you to be more productive, more social, more successful and happier all around."

Maybe the answers to your "whys" will be different. Maybe you want to feel more confident. Maybe you want to lower your lipid panel and lighten the load on your heart so that, one day, you can attend your baby's graduation. Whatever your answers, by homing in on your deep-down whys, you give that couch and a pizza a run for their money. **Whatever is tempting you from doing what you know is right, ask yourself:**

What's my why? Because the why—or the *who* you're doing it for—can help force the how.

"I'm thankful for being diagnosed with diabetes this year because it finally solved a problem I've been struggling with for seven years," says Tina Tessina, PhD, a psychotherapist in Southern California, and author of *Money, Sex, and Kids*, who was eating a healthy vegetarian diet and exercising, but still couldn't budge some extra weight. Then, "blood tests showed I had entered into diabetes II levels," says Tessina. Eager for more information, she began taking classes through her health insurer and learned about counting carbohydrates and the plate method (filling a plate with half unstarchy vegetables, one-quarter protein, and one-quarter starches), and "I began losing weight," says Tessina. "It was amazingly easy. I've gotten my blood sugar under control through diet and no medication." Her diagnosis was a "why" that made her dig deeper and discover the power of a low-carbohydrate diet. And if she's tempted to fall into her former habits, her success with her health is a "why" that can keep her on point.

Tessina's "why" is saving her life, and when you trace back what you're doing to its core, it can help push you through the tough times, too. Why are you rushing to a meeting, running on a treadmill, researching doctors, and writing all those thank-you notes? To show you care, to succeed in your dreams, to make your mother proud, to make yourself proud, to live a long, healthy life. Put *your* answer to your whys on a sticky note and paste it on your computer, then don't take your eye off that prize.

And you know what? Sometimes asking yourself "why"

reveals surprising results. Sometimes the why turns out not to be worth it. And sometimes the project—learning a language, training for a marathon—is the why itself, for it challenges your mind or proves you can do it. "I'm all for rewards," says New York stress management specialist Debbie Mandel, "but I think sometimes we need to see the reward we get by *doing* the project. Having a glass of wine or chocolate as a reward is fine, but it's not connected to *why* you want to get your paper done. I think there are rewards in completion and seeing the results. A job well done *is* a reward."

The why is the point of it all—of life, love, and happiness. Ask yourself that question, and be bold enough to answer.

Park the car or drive away.

The other day, a white construction van pulled up outside my home office window and sat, its engine idling for fifteen irritating minutes before it finally pulled away. Two days later, Gus and I were sitting outside at a French café in town when a car pulled up at the curb and sat with its engine running for half an hour until the driver finally turned it off and got out of the car. The idling, in both cases, drove me absolutely bananas.

Yes, part of the reason is that the smell of exhaust fills the air, and the sound of the engine punctures the peace, but an idling car also seems on edge: We don't know how long the car is going to be there, and apparently, neither does the car. All in all, it's a perfect metaphor for that awful feeling we get in life limbo. **If you're torn between two choices, your indecision is as loud an *emotional* noise as an eighteen-wheeler idling in front of you.** The air you're breathing is thick as smoke, half breaths full of stress and strain. Like the famously indecisive Hamlet who couldn't answer himself "To be or not to be," we owe it to ourselves the gift of a decision: Either park the car or drive away.

When I met Jen, a young mom, she was torn about whether to keep her work-at-home job or find something else. The logistics of the job were perfect for raising her young daughter, but the work wasn't fulfilling her, and the energy she was wasting on her idling between the options was exhausting her! I helped her decide that, for six months, she'd park the car. "Once I decided I was going to stay put for six solid months," says Jen, "I was able to do my job and appreciate the time it gave me with my daughter and husband." By parking the car, she could enjoy her life for a minute without the hum of uncertainty echoing in her head like a car engine. And a few months from now, she'll see how she feels at the curb.

My friend Phillip, on the other hand, was fighting with his girlfriend because they didn't seem to be on the same page. For six months, he idled. "I'm tired of trying," he finally told me. "I want to just *be*." And while it wasn't easy to let go, he put in the keys and drove away to find a woman who wanted what he did in love.

You deserve to feel settled in one way or another. Give yourself that chance. Either turn off the car and exhale in peace, or drive away and see what's out there. How do you know which way to go? Well, review your routes and see which road seems smoother.

If you park the car—you stay in your job or relationship or home—is there something you can do that will make it better? Maybe, by making small changes in yourself or your environment, you can make parking the car feel like a brand-new, brighter experience. If you drive away—you leave your job or relationship or home—do you have a plan where you'll go next? Can you handle the uncertainty of not knowing, or the potential disappointment if you find yourself still driving a year from now? Maybe you have it in you, a desire to try new things and a confidence that no matter what you find on the road ahead, it will be better than what you have now.

Either way, make a decision. Life in limbo will kill your spirit, sap your energy, and add stress you don't need. So either shut off the ignition and lock it up, or roll down the windows and get going on the highway of life. Stop idly "trying" to make both sides work or both choices possible. Park the car or drive away so you, too, can just be.

....

Use your underdog as an upper hand.

....

Sometimes, the lower you are on your ladder in life, the better off you are; with less to lose, you have much more to gain. And no one learns that lesson better than the underdog. Take, for example, the victory of the San Francisco Giants in the 2010 World Series that no one—aside from devoted Giants fans—expected them to win. Yet as closing pitcher Brian "The Beard" Wilson explained on *The Tonight Show*, that's one of the reasons they *did*.

"There's a lot of hype in baseball," Wilson said, "and if you're at the top, you can only go down. So going in as the underdog, I mean, we're *supposed* to lose, right? So, let's *not* lose, and let's show them what we're about." The team that was supposed to lose beat the overwhelming favorite Texas Rangers 3–1 to take the World Series title.

The fact is, being the underdog can give you the upper hand. How? Well, when you're not in the running for the title, you can take the competition out of the equation and just be your best you. Think: *If I'm going to go down, then I'll go down being the best, most authentic version of me possible*. Work from your heart, date from your heart, speak from your heart, write from your heart. I've seen more contestants on *American Idol* rock it out when they choose to ignore the battle for supremacy and just do what they did best. **When you're feeling low, remember: Being an underdog gives you the upper hand. Without the pressure to be number one, you can just be number *you*.**

You don't need to write the best proposal that's ever been written, you just need to write one that gets the point across. You don't need to completely ace your speech, you just need to get through it respectably. You don't need to be madly, wildly in love with your partner again by the end of the getaway weekend, you just need to like each other more than you did last Wednesday. Sometimes, life is like picking a price for the Showcase Showdown on *The Price Is Right*: If your opponent says $19,000 and the actual price is more than that, you can win by saying $19,001. So don't make the road ahead of you seem bigger than it is. Just walk your walk, talk your talk, and do the best you can.

When you're at the bottom of the canyon, you don't have anywhere to go but up. So take a deep breath, steel yourself, and start climbing. Believe in yourself and do the best you can, and you just may end up succeeding while doing it.

Without self-confidence and faith in yourself, the more you'll lose and the more you'll fear you'll *continue* to. But every underdog victory that's ever been turned into a made-for-TV movie can remind you otherwise: Being on the bottom isn't a sign that you'll lose again. It's a call to win. It's a call to remember that when the pressure is off to ace it, you can pull out the best in yourself and show everyone what you can do. So why not pull out the stops and surprise them all? There's a reason everyone roots for the underdog: because we've all struggled up from the bottom at some point. Which is why when the less likely one wins—hello, highlight reel!—it's the most thrilling type of victory there is.

Let it go like a Chinese lantern.

I don't ski. There, I've said it.

Growing up, I skied about once a year working my way up from beginner slopes to the intermediate ones. Then, some years ago, I went to the Sundance Film Festival in Park City, Utah, where some friends had invited me to stay in their chalet. The first morning, we met for a morning ski—where I learned fast that the bunny slopes in Utah are like the black diamonds of the hills I knew in New Jersey. So I snowplowed down a few paths and was relieved when it was time to ski home. Not only was it our last run, but what a posh entrance into the house, right? Well. Then I saw the incline of the final trail, which seemed dangerous to peer *over*, let alone set off down it on slidely things! Apparently, people who rent chalets you have to ski into are all, like, really good skiers.

Still, I tried. But terrified and whimpering every time I gained speed, I finally took off my skis and clomped sideways down the hill. Ten minutes after the others had swooshed to the door, I showed up with the skis in my arms and tears staining my face—not such a posh entrance, after all. But once I started laughing off the embarrassment, I embraced what it gave me. Because that was the day I let the illusion go. Me? I don't downhill ski. I'll cross-country ski through the woods and meet y'all back at the house for hot chocolate in front of the fire, but you won't see me heading toward the big slope. I'm not a skier. And I feel so free saying that.

A disaster isn't always a disaster. Sometimes, it's a gift. Take what feels like a moment of defeat and see it as an epiphany, for if nothing else, it's a freeing symbol that you are not meant to be doing it. Or buying it. Or playing that sport. Or marrying that person. Sometimes, finding out you loathe a career or a camera or a relationship is a very freeing thing. I picture it like the tradition of the Chinese lanterns.

In Eastern Asia, there is a tradition of making wishes, lighting lanterns, then letting them go into the night sky or setting them out onto the water. In a way, it's a gesture of letting your wants go and giving in to the power of the universe. Well, you can let your defeats go in the same way. Consider seeing your setback as a symbolic end of one well-tried path and the bright beginning of a new one. Yes, there's something to be said for sticking with things and pushing past struggles until you come out on the other side; but there's also a time for waving the white flag, lying back on the lounger, and freeing yourself up to figure out what it is you like *more*.

If you've tried everything from vinyasa to bikram to power sessions of downward dog and *still* hate yoga? Let it go and free yourself to find a movement you love. If your fourth date doesn't feel any more comfortable than the first, let it go and thank the happy hour gods you don't have to try it again. If you've been trying to sort your own taxes or fix your own roof or color your own hair and keep running into walls of frustration or failure? Let it go; you can hire people for those things and free yourself up to learn what you're better at.

My friend Christine spent years building her résumé to get

into the grad school program for public policy at a prestigious university, then, two weeks into class realized she *hated* it. Was it hard to face her feelings of failure, her family and friends' reactions, and the lost years and money she'd put into her plan? Yes. But while she didn't know what she wanted to do with her life instead, she sure knew one thing she *didn't*. So Christine let her lantern go, dropped out of school, started over, and now excels in her work in corporate training in a way she never would have on her prior path.

People change, wants change, needs change. And like a closet with only enough room for a certain number of clothes, we have to let some things go to let the new things into our lives. Don't let a defeat beat you. See it as a sign of new things to come. Light your lantern, raise the flame above your head, and say good-bye to your struggle of trying so hard to make something work. Feel as free as a lantern floating into the night sky, ready to land at the dawn of something new.

Get the ball in the basket.

I've come to love the NBA. Maybe it's because my husband plies me with delectable head rubs through the second half of big games (and now he gets one every time I watch a decidedly un-guycentric show). But I still get a kick out of it when players are asked about their strategy and say they just want to go out there and "get the ball in the basket."

Oh wow, we think, *that's some strategy*. But guess what? It *is*. In sports, like in life, sometimes we forget that the whole thing is really as simple as that. Yes, in basketball, you also need to maximize your rebounding, increase the ball movement, bolster your defense, maybe double-team their key players (I'm not kidding, I really do love it.); but what it all comes down to—when you add up those points and crown a winner—is how many balls went through that hoop. "The end result might be that it's not a dunk at the end, but it might be a layup, which still counts for two points," said Phoenix Suns coach Alvin Gentry in 2009, after losing superstar player Amar'e Stoudemire to the Knicks. "It might not be one of the Amar'e *SportsCenter* dunks," said Gentry, "but if we can get it in the basket, then that's what we're going to try to do."

The same goes for life: When you're feeling pressured by the first step of a big project, the first day on a new job, or the first date with a new person, don't let yourself get ten steps ahead, or wrapped up in red tape, logistics, nerves, or big strategies. Take it one day at a time, one date at a time, or one step at a time. Focusing on the simplest, purest goal can lighten the load you carry and smooth out the path to get there. **In your own way—in your project, your pitch, your performance—aim to achieve your purest goal, pared down to its essence: Aim to get *your* ball in the basket.**

So what's your ball and where's your basket? Well, give yourself a press conference and find out. Ask yourself just that: *What's my basket? And how do I get the ball in?*

If you've run up your credit cards? Spend less, pay off your debt more. If you're still stuck on perfecting the first page of your business plan? Skip to page two and *get writing*. If you're not feeling loved? Become a kind, loving person and see what you attract in return. Anytime you feel stalled by size or strategy or long-term goals, pare your situation down to the smallest denominator, its purest form. Allow yourself the gift of forgetting the complications and future next steps for a minute, because if you can find the simplest way to look at your situation, you'll clarify your path, which will make you more likely to get going on it.

Aim, shoot, score. Get your own ball in, one basket at a time.

Break the un-rules!

When screenwriter Charlie Kaufman was hired to adapt author Susan Orlean's book *The Orchid Thief* for the big screen, he struggled trying to find a way to bring the nonfiction title to life. So he broke the rules—well, the "rules" other people seemed to follow anyway. Instead of predictably adapting the book, he created a meta-take *about* his experience adapting the book. And in 2002, the film *Adaptation* received an Oscar nomination for Best Writing (Adapted Screenplay). Kaufman simply wasn't getting anywhere doing it how it had always been done. So he forged his own way.

Maybe you can do the same. Sometimes, it's not only okay to break the rules, it's healthy! Because not all rules are even "rules" at all. So take an un-rule and break it.

That's how I got out of a funk on a recent vacation. Our final morning in Costa Rica, Gus and I rented two bikes from our hotel and pedaled to a beautiful black sand beach. Five minutes after settling down on our towels with our books, it started to rain—we're talking *buckets*. All I could think was that our last lazy day of vacation was ruined.

But as we ran for cover at a little restaurant overlooking the water, we took in our situation. I mean, we were in Costa Rica, for goodness' sake! So while life had changed the rules on us, we could change the rules right back.

Even though it was only eleven a.m., we ordered two Pilsen beers. And even though it was a public place, we kicked off our flip-flops, racked up the billiard balls, and played a few games of pool barefoot on the wooden floor, dancing to Latin music through the downpour. Two hours later, though, the rain was still falling in sheets.

"How long do you think we'll have to wait until the rain stops?" I asked Gus.

"Why do we have to wait until the rain stops?" he asked.

"Uh," I said, "because you don't ride bicycles in the rain?"

Gus shrugged, asked the manager for a plastic bag, and wrapped our things tightly inside. Then we hopped on our bikes and broke the un-rules by riding barefoot back to town, steering around chickens and whizzing through puddles on the muddy dirt roads. *He's right*, I thought. *Why* can't *you ride bicycles in the rain?* That wonderful wet day is still one we talk about most.

So break the un-rules in your own way. Go for a swim five minutes after you eat. Wear white after Labor Day. Drink your red wine cold. Brainstorm ideas in the bathtub. Or stick to your healthy eating plan by walking around the house in a bikini (that's a great technique, by the way—it works for me).

As Emerson once wrote, "Do not go where the path may lead; go, instead, where there is no path, and leave a trail." The more you embrace what works best for you, the happier you'll be. Don't worry about how other people work or date or exercise. **Don't just take a number, fill out the forms, and color inside the lines. Be creative, productive, and happy in the best ways you know how.** And if that means wearing a pair of big, fuzzy bear slippers while you work, have at it.

Elbow fear out of the way.

It was time for the celebratory toast at my friend's wedding ten years ago when Dave, the best man, could not be found. We all knew he was a little nervous about giving his speech, but we didn't know *how* nervous until they stalled the proceedings and a pal went to fetch him. That's when he discovered Dave huddled in a bathroom stall, covered—face, neck, and arms—with hives. The groom's uncle stepped in and gave the speech instead, and Dave slinked back into the reception about an hour later saying, "See? I told you I'd be scared." That's fear for ya. And it holds us back from so many rewarding experiences.

We're afraid we'll be turned down, so we don't ask. We're afraid someone won't like our song, so we don't play it. We're afraid to be thought foolish, so we don't ask questions. We're afraid we'll be bad at explaining it, so we don't stand up and try. Well, here's a different idea: Let's show fear what we're made of and give ourselves a chance to see what we can do. Those knots of fear? Elbow it out of the way and push past it.

The next time you're at a party and see someone you wish you had the guts to talk to, don't spend the night grabbing stuffed mushrooms as they come out of the catering door (though it *is* a good trick, right?). Go for it. Give that fear a good jab in the gut and talk to them. Because facing a fear brings reward no matter what. You'll be rewarded with success or you'll be rewarded with pride that you tried. **Either way, you win. Because conquering fear reaches greater heights on the curves of life than failing reaches the lows.**

In a film created by the founders of the Good Men Project, father Stuart Horwitz tells of taking his daughter Fifer out "busking"—playing guitar and singing songs for cash on street corners. While some people didn't like the idea, Stuart felt that having her play music in front of a crowd who hasn't asked you to be there was helping build his daughter's self-esteem. As he said in the film, "The other side of fear is a blissful self-confidence you have to earn, you can't buy." I think all of us—old or young, settled or searching—can remind ourselves of the same thing.

Hey, rejection happens. But don't reject *yourself* before giving someone the chance to. Don't strip yourself of experiences and possible success because you're afraid it won't work out. NBC's *Parenthood* may have said it best: "Life will knock you down more times than you can possibly imagine. Don't knock *yourself* down." Yeah, you might fall or fail. But you might *not*. Don't let fear hold you back on the dock worrying what will happen if you stand up on the water skis; elbow it out of the way and try the ride.

Whether you succeed or fail, when you put yourself out there, you win. You win with success in your endeavor or with satisfaction and a blissful self-confidence you couldn't have earned any other way. Don't let fear take a prize like that away from you.

Keep going, keep gunning.

Think it's too late for something you want to pursue? Let me tell you the story of movie director David Wain.

He directed his first feature, *Wet Hot American Summer*, in 2001, and although the film has gained a cult following, it did poorly at the box office. So David spent six years writing treatments, pitching ideas, developing stories, and taking meetings to get a new project going. Finally, he got his break.

"I got a script written by someone I knew that was being set up at a studio," says David. "It was exactly my sensibility and I knew I could nail it." Oh, and the production company executive? A former agent of David's, who was rooting for him.

David got a meeting with the head of the studio to pitch himself as director, and spent a month creating storyboards and casting and music ideas in a big presentation binder. Then he bought a ticket to L.A. "I knew at very least," he says, "I'd give them a killer sell and be on the studio's radar." But as David was walking through the studio lot, he got a call from his agent.

"Your meeting is canceled," his agent said. "They gave the job to someone else."

David, stunned, retreated to his rental car. "I looked in the mirror at myself, devastated," he says. "And then I thought, 'I'm not gonna quit doing this. This is what I do. And if I can keep going after this, I know I'll never quit.'"

Somehow, he says, it was a liberating commitment. And he stuck with it. He's since directed films including *Role Models* and *Wanderlust*—and there's truly no end in sight.

David's story is a lesson for us all. If your passion for your dream is a force that moves you, keep going and keep gunning. It is never too late to be the person you want to be. In job, in spirit, in love, in what you create or who you can become. Just set your sights and stay the course. Like the words attributed to author George Eliot, "It's never too late to be who you might have been."

If you want to change careers, you can. If you want to fall in love, you can. If you want to travel the world, set a swimming record, write your memoirs, learn to blow glass, or start your own business, you *can*. **There are people out there, every day, starting fresh or starting over. There is no age limit on dreams.** If you believe in yourself and what you can do, you can make it happen. And as scientist Barbara McClintock knew, that's true even if people don't think what you're doing is worth it.

McClintock studied chromosomes in maize for forty years,

and though she was largely ignored for much of her work at the time, she was eventually awarded the Nobel Prize in Medicine in 1983—fifty-six long, tedious years after she earned her PhD and began her research. McClintock is now credited as the discoverer of transposable genes, which is the basis for today's research in genetic engineering. Time and age simply can't compete with passion.

So don't let what's been done before hold you back from what you try. You can have the love and the life of your dreams if you believe in it enough to pursue it. David did. Barbara did. And you should, too. Keep going, keep gunning, and don't let anyone get in your way.

....

Appreciate your abundance.

....

I don't know about you, but I get "order envy" in restaurants. Just when I've finished debating four delicious options and finally feel good about what I'm getting, I see the steak on someone else's plate and wish I'd gotten that instead. Life is the very same way: It's sometimes hard to feel satisfied with what's on our plates when we see what someone else has. And yet, when it comes down to it, we're swimming in abundance.

Our desires are relative. In one famous study out of the Harvard School of Public Health, participants were asked if they'd rather make $50,000 in a society where others earned $25,000, or make $100,000 where others earned $200,000.

The results? Fifty-six percent of people chose the former. Think about that: More people would take *half* the money just to feel richer in comparison, to have a leg up on everyone else. So if you want to feel happier, **the key is not in actually having the most toys, but *feeling* like you have plenty. What really matters in your life may already be there.**

So the next time you find yourself feeling cheated, left behind, or just plain less than anyone else, focus on what is full in your life. If you have a safe and secure home, you are abundantly sheltered. If you have food to eat for dinner, you are abundantly fed. If you have shoes and clothes for your body, you are abundantly dressed. If you have a family or friends who care for you, you are abundantly loved. All that other stuff? It's extra. That flat-screen TV and the sushi dinner where you splurged—again—on the yellowtail and jalapeno with ponzu sauce because it's so good how can you not? It's great, but it's extra. It doesn't matter what other people have when you have everything you need.

When I visited Samoa, a stunning country of small islands in the South Pacific where even the police wear sarongs as their uniforms, I noticed that while they lived one of the most unmaterialistic lifestyles, they also seemed like some of the happiest people. The Fa'asamoa, their way of life, is based around villages of traditional brightly painted *fale* homes: open wood-floored structures without walls or windows, where women weave on the floor inside with fresh frangipani flowers in their hair and families play volleyball together in the front yard. Yes, they live along stunning reef-protected turquoise waters, but where were their five-bedroom, three-bath Mc-Mansions with Sub-Zero fridges and BMW convertibles?

"We have everything we need here," said resident Kristian Louiz Saitofiga Lam-Scanlan. "We have land and the ocean. Fish is free if you fish for it yourself. The only reason you starve is if you don't work to get it." So simple and so happy. They only work as long as they have to so they can spend the rest of their time swimming and eating long, lingering Sunday meals steamed over umu ovens. They've found abundance in having just what they need and making the most of it, and so can all of us.

Actively appreciate the abundance in your life. Look around whatever room you're in and see how full of abundance your life is right now. Maybe you're holding a cup of hot Starbucks (extra) between checking emails on your iPhone (definitely extra) before heading to meet your friends for cocktails (now that's just gravy). You have life, fresh air, food to eat, water to drink, and people to share your abundance and good health. You have the seeds of an extraordinary life; you have everything you need.

....

Walk a positive tightrope.

....

Derren Brown is a performer in England who combines the powers of suggestion and psychology into his act in order to, as he says, "seemingly predict and control human behavior."

On one episode of his TV series *Trick or Treat*, he conducted an experiment in negative suggestion in which he visited the high-wire artist Henry at Zippos circus in the UK. Henry was famous for skipping rope on a tightrope and had never, as Derren said, fallen off doing that trick. But what would happen if Derren put Henry's positive thoughts to the test? "The thought, *I must try not to fall*," said Derren, "is precisely the *wrong* way to think thirty feet up in the air on a high wire, even if you're the world's best at it." So that's just the thought he put into Henry's head.

"Focus on *not* wobbling and *not* falling off," he told Henry, who was about to step out onto the wire. "Just make sure you *don't* wobble and fall off." As Derren put it, "The instruction 'Try not to fall off,' residently delivered, is amplified by the inflation of an air bag . . . Henry's unconscious is, for the first time, thinking in terms of, 'I mustn't fall off,' which can only take him one way." It did. Henry fell from the high wire into the air bag and seemed visibly shaken by the whole experience.

Now, I do take the performance with a grain of salt as this was all for television, but similar incidents have happened to me. When I took my first surfing lesson in Maui a few years ago, I was a wreck when I paddled out thinking, *I hope I don't wipe out! I hope I don't get hurt!* Yet when I was told to focus on standing up and smiling for a camera on shore with my best "hang ten" pose? I stood and surfed in tall and proud. Sure, I was on three feet of calm water riding six-inch waves after a push-off by my instructor, but still. **Whether we're trying to balance on an object or trying to balance in life, we will only**

succeed if we're focused on succeeding. If we focus on trying not to fail, fall, or lose, we might end up doing just that.

Avoid negative suggestion by walking a positive line. If you're about to give a big speech, instead of thinking, *I hope I don't blow this,* think about what you *want* to happen, like, *I want to get my message out, inspire them, and be myself while doing it.* And if you want to do well pitching your ideas to your boss, instead of thinking, *I hope she doesn't regret hiring me,* think about what you *want* to happen, like, *I want to tell her all the ideas I brainstormed, so that even if my boss doesn't like them, she'll respect me for getting creative outside the box.*

When I was single, I often found myself thinking, *I'm sick and tired of being single,* which unconsciously created a negative cycle in my dating life that attracted, well, more situations that made me feel sick and tired. So, I changed my mind-set. Every morning, I got excited and hopeful about meeting someone smart, fun, and just right for me. Eight months after embracing my "dating optimism," I ran into my now-husband Gus, who was all the positive things I'd focused on. I was so floored by the effects of my positive thinking that I wrote about my experience and the specific strategies that worked in *Meeting Your Half-Orange: An Utterly Upbeat Guide to Using Dating Optimism to Find Your Perfect Match.*

The point is, you'll get what you think about, and you'll head where your head is at. It's how our minds and bodies work. So stop giving your focus to what you *don't* want in life and start talking about what you *do*: Ask for positive, inspiring moments. Ask to win the point, complete the race, keep it up, and stay on course. Ask to stand up, stay tall, balance, and thrive. Ask for love and friendship and respect and success, for good luck and abundance and bliss. Then, when you step onto the tightrope of life, you'll be primed to stand tall and succeed.

Take back control.

Have you ever had one of those "falling" dreams? They're terrifying. Because the feeling of losing control in any form can send us reeling. Which is how Eva Wisnik found her life's greatest lesson in her hardest year.

"The year 2009 was the suckiest year in the universe for me," said Wisnik, if she may be so blunt. That's the year the business at her thirteen-year-old time management training and placement firm in New York fell by 80 percent. "I had never in fourteen years ever felt like I had no control," said Wisnik, "but there was nothing I could do that would make the business come back." So, she aimed to gain back her confidence by challenging herself in other ways. "Since I wasn't getting the intellectual challenge," Wisnik told me, "I decided to do all these physical things." In one year, she went parachuting and trapeze flying and hired a rock-climbing instructor to teach her how to scale big red boulders out West. So though she was stalled in her business life, she says, "I felt like I was still moving forward."

It's a wonderful lesson: **If you're feeling a loss of control in**

one part of your life, find a way to gain it in another. Even if it's just in an eight-foot-square area of your home or office.

An old boss of mine gave me advice for those days at work when you can't seem to muster up the mind you need: Clean out your desk. After two hours of tossing out old sugar packets and putting your paperclips in one clean place, you'll find yourself feeling ready to tackle your work again. In the same way, when your personal life feels heavy, clear your physical space: tidy your closet and clean under your bed and you'll start feeling lighter in your body, too. As Dr. Drew Pinsky suggested to a patient feeling a lack of love on one episode of VH1's *Celebrity Rehab*, controlling what you *can* will make you feel better about what you can't. "Emptiness is a hard one to fix," said Dr. Drew. "I would suggest you start simple. Clean your room. Get out of bed . . . Own your environment, own your life."

Harnessing control, as it turns out, is a key to happiness. In humans and animals, "loss of control can be very stresssful," Bruce Hood, PhD, founder of the Bristol Cognitive Development Centre in England, told me. "That's why we prefer predictability. The brain is always seeking out order and structure in a world of uncertainty and ambiguity." So when the rug of control is pulled out from under you, reach up and grasp order and structure in some other way.

You are not a small pawn in the random roll of life. You *have* control in more areas of your life than you don't. But it is up to you to grab it. Take back the wheel, hold tight, and steer your own route in whatever way you can.

....

Focus on the horizon.

....

When I first moved to Venice Beach with Gus, my friend Suyai said she had two pieces of advice for me: "One, get a bike with gears," she said. "And two, whenever you feel stressed, go to the beach until you're not stressed anymore."

After a few months of happily shifting into high gear on my bike, I found myself in a state of panic over trying to complete a work project. As I paced my house, nearly hyperventilating over the fact that I was certain I'd never get it done, I heard my friend Suyai's voice in my head. So I rode to the beach in low gear and put my bare feet in the water.

Standing at the foot of nature's majesty, my breathing slowed, my muscles relaxed, and my mind stopped racing. And seeing the size of that ocean, the endless crash of those waves that had been moving millions of years before I got there and—God willing—would be moving for millions more, I realized how small and surmountable my problems were in comparison. Yes, for this week of my life, the work project was a big deal. But seeing that ocean reminded me that this was just one week of my long life, which was just a wink of a moment on Earth. The horizon steadied me. **It's much like the advice for seasickness: If you're feeling sick from the rocking motion at your feet, you focus on the steady horizon in the distance.** Because nature's horizon, its inveterate sunrises and sunsets, the evolution of a planet that changes so slowly over time, is a reminder that our issues in this life *can* be handled.

And you can experience some of that same power of nature by bringing the outside in. A 1984 study by behavioral scientist Roger Ulrich at Texas A&M University found that patients in hospitals who could see trees from their windows had improved recovery rates and fewer post-surgical complications than those facing a brick wall. In another study, Ulrich found that, by adding flowers and plants to an office, men generated 15 percent more ideas and women found more creative and flexible ideas to problems.

So adjust your view from inside so that you can see trees, plants, or flowers outside. Or buy an indoor-friendly peace lily, African violet, or a philodendron, with bright green leaves that can withstand a few days without water while you spend a weekend in the water. Watching plants bloom and grow is a reminder that life is so much bigger than us, that the daily stress we create for ourselves doesn't add up to much in the grand scheme of life.

Let nature and the horizon realign your view so what you're dealing with now feels more manageable. Walk in the woods or hike up a mountain. Find a vista to view the sunset or an open field in the dark of night. Observe the orchid on your table about to burst to life. Head to an ocean and watch the waves turn rocks into sand. The bigger a view you can get of the earth ahead of you, the smaller your problems can be measured in comparison.

Take the big view. Let the horizon steady you.

When Your
RELATIONSHIPS
Could Use a Reboot . . .

Enjoy the cusp!

If all we lived for were the big moments in life—the announcement, the speech, the win, the promotion—we'd really be losing out on some of the good stuff. Because the truth is, those moments just before we reach our goals in life, work, and love are often more special than the moments we achieve them. I'm talking about the cusp. Like the tantalizing aroma of coffee before you take your first sip, the cusp of a big moment is part of what makes the moment so big in the first place. That cusp—that point of intersection between the anticipation of something happening and it coming to fruition—is everything.

What, after all, is a first kiss without the uncertain seconds just before your lips meet? Those seconds are the ones charged with energy, nervousness, and hope. The cusp is us holding our breath as the quarterback throws the touchdown pass, us tingling with anticipation as the drumroll begins, us counting how many names are left before the one we know is handed the diploma, us gasping before the trapeze artist grabs the bar. What, after all, is the moment most brides talk about before their wedding? Not the part of exchanging rings, reciting vows, or even the first kiss as a married couple; it's the moment of walking down the aisle *toward* those big moments. The cusp, you see, is everything.

There's optimism in the cusp: We're trusting that the moments will follow through and turn out well. And when they do, we can collapse into it, even more grateful. So perhaps it's time to start appreciating the cusp of great things as much as we appreciate the moments themselves. In life, in love. Yes, getting the job, graduating the program, and falling in love are wonderful, and if you do them right, they are all they're cracked up to be. **But where would the greatness of the good things be without the cusp of buildup just before you get there?**

Make it your goal to appreciate the moment you're in now rather than peering ahead into the future. Ask yourself: What's great about your life right now, a life that will change when you reach your destination? What can you smile about today? And who is around you, supporting your journey? Feel grateful for all of it, because this moment is as special as the one you'll have when you get there.

Enjoy the cusp of eating a dessert as your fork cuts into a piece of cake and your mouth opens in expectation. Love the cusp of a bursting flower bud about to bloom, which can be as beautiful as the bloom itself. And what about the thrilling cusp of a big drop on a roller coaster—those moments when the sounds of the clicking train are replaced with a deafening silence, when your giddy fear turns to panic before you swoop down the hill? The seconds before the drop are as exhilarating as dropping down the hill itself.

If you're desperately hoping for the next big place in your life to arrive, yes, you should think about the future and focus on what you want, but don't forget to love and appreciate the fleeting place you're in *this moment*. Life moves quickly, changes happen, and love surprises you. Don't forget to enjoy the cusp right now, before you miss it.

Feel warmth within the quills.

My husband doesn't leave the toilet seat up or the cap off the toothpaste. But he does other things. Like, say, when he comes in from being out, he likes to turn on all the overhead lights like a trail of Hansel and Gretel's breadcrumbs through the house. And he likes to leave an aluminum can on the counter just eleven inches from—but not in—the recycling bin. And there is an issue with the toothpaste, actually: He squeezes it out all cockamamie, like it's been run over by a golf cart, which takes my tube flattening back to square one every morning. And while I do find these things a little grating at times, I also remember something else: When I was single, my home was always exactly as I'd left it, yet I yearned for someone I loved in the house with me: someone to turn the lights on, to leave a can around now and then, to mess with the bathroom sink.

So when I need to see the bright side, I look at that gnarled toothpaste tube as a reminder that my dream came true and that if the cost of love is dealing with a few puny habits, I was in. In fact, I started to look at each of those shining overhead lights not as irritations, but as reminders of him in our home, of Gus's untold way of saying, "I love you." Of course, I made the mistake of *telling* him this, and now every time I groan and shut off a light, he grins and says, "See how much I love you?" Still, it helps.

When you're ready to curse the way the towels are folded or the direction the toilet paper is rolling (or that the roll is sitting on the floor instead of, ahem, on the dispenser where it should be), remind yourself that in the bigger picture, there is love. There is love to help you muss up the bed, run the gas down in the car, and leave all the cupboard doors open; another being who's chosen to share space and time with you. **Little aggravations are a small price to pay for a partner in crime on the journey of life.**

It's like the story of the porcupines that dates back to the German philosopher and infamous pessimist Arthur Schopenhauer; he was said to have not seen the positive message, but as with everything in life, there is a more positive side, if you look for it. As the tale goes, it was a cold, cold winter. Lots of animals couldn't handle the freeze and died. But the shivering porcupines, determined to live, decided that if they grouped together, they could protect themselves and keep warm. The problem? As soon as they got close enough to get warm, the pain of the quills hurt too much. But when the porcupines separated, they became so cold that they began to die, lonely and frozen. The porcupines had to make a choice: They could either accept the poking painful quills of their companions or die off one by one. They agreed: It was better to be warm and live together than die apart and alone.

Now, not everyone wants a relationship and might prefer to be alone—and unlike these porcupines, you won't die from it! You can, of course, live a vibrant full life on your own. But in every relationship in your life—with a romantic partner, your friends, your family—there *will* be quills. In a happy relationship, you simply must learn to live with the little stuff and focus on the warm, wonderful qualities instead—the ones that *really* matter. For me, Gus and I still talk into the night, spend hours perfecting a vat of gumbo, and he keeps me laughing in line at the grocery store.

Maybe your partner is messy and you're neat, or they want to blast Led Zeppelin in the car while you'd prefer Liszt. Those quills will bug and hurt you from time to time, no question. But if the other stuff is there—the things that make you feel loved and smart and sexy and valued and funny and on a shared path to a wonderful future—that's the warmth. And *that's* what matters.

....

Be your own gift-with-purchase.

....

Somewhere along the line of relationships, we've come to look to our partners to give us every single thing we want: A confidant. A cohort. Comic relief. Sexual pleasure. The perfect social companion. And how about a few bonus gifts-with-purchase—like season tickets, a boat in the marina, or an "in" at Louis Vuitton with a personal discount.

It's like a shortcut to getting everything we want in one easy package. In some ways, we're projecting what we wish for ourselves: We want someone successful so we can feel like we are, someone creative because we wish we were more so, or someone adventurous because we wish we leapt without a net. Whatever our reasons, if the partners or spouses we've already chosen don't have all those qualities or gifts, we're disappointed and can, over time, grow resentful for it.

How about this instead: **How about we become the people with qualities we wish our mates had? Instead of expecting your relationship or friendships to give it all to you, give what you can to yourself. Be your *own* gift-with-purchase.**

Lest you think I'm telling you to settle in life or love, let me explain. I tell singles to "ask for it all!" and I believe that you should. But by "it all" I mean the big things: feeling loved, respected, smart, funny, and—in the case of a romantic partnership—hot as heck. What I don't mean by "it all": someone who likes the same toppings on a pizza, knows every word to all the same albums, or is equally charming with every relative you have. If you score on one of these points: bonus! But rather than expecting your partner or best friend to fill every exact box that you do, remember: That's what social circles are for. And that's what you as an individual are for: Be your *own* gift-with-purchase.

Forget expecting a partner who lives to travel so you'll have an impetus to leave town: Get traveling on your own! Forget expecting a partner who shakes it on the dance floor; sign up with an eager friend or learn the two-step on your own some Tuesday night. Forget expecting a partner to be wildly successful: Become wildly successful yourself! Each of us can be strong and fearless and successful in our own right, so why are we letting ourselves be suckered by our subconscious and seeking out *mates* who have those qualities instead? Be the happy, fulfilled person you want to be all on your own.

And of course by being your *own* gift-with-purchase, you'll attract the very partner, friends, and career you wanted in the first place. And like the "free gift" you get with your infomercial purchase, you have to admit, that's a darn good deal.

Just do you.

Many years ago, I was asked to write a story for a magazine I respected so much that I worried if I was worthy enough to be printed in its pages. So while I accepted the assignment, I spent the first three days frozen in fear, debating if I should bow out.

I don't know how to write like the stories I've seen, I thought, biting my nails and brainstorming how I might change my writing style to please the politicians who read it. And that's when I realized my job wasn't to mimic other people; my job was to write like *me.* And if they didn't like it, they just wouldn't ask me to write for them again, right? Well, they liked the story and they did ask me to write for them again. But it was a nerve-wrangling experience that changed me forever. For in our insecure moments, the only thing we can do is turn to a true confidence in who we are. As music mogul Russell Simmons advises in *Do You!,* his bestselling book, just, well, *do you.*

The next time you're nervous before a speech, a date, an interview, or an assignment, direct your beating heart and shaking hands to a more positive place, by remembering that a rush of nerves is similar to what you feel when you're excited. "Nervousness can be a negative or a positive," TV producer Mark Burnett said to finalist Kristina Kuzmic-Crocco on *Your OWN Show,* who was gunning for her own program on Oprah Winfrey's OWN. "The positive can turn nervousness into excitement," said Burnett. "It's the same feeling. Think about it: It's a physiological feeling. You decide which one it is. Make it excitement."

And what is there to be excited about? Knowing you're there to do you. **Only you have your life experience, your point of view, and your voice. And you'll only succeed by being the truest, most authentic version of you.** You're the only one who can talk, smile, or tell a story as you would. Just do what you know how to do, say what you know how to say, and express yourself in your own unique way, then let life make the decision from there. Don't try to be the person you think other people expect you to be. The truth is, your audience hopes and expects only one thing: *for you to do you.*

You think you're not funny enough? Smart enough? Polished enough? Pretty enough? Or, in my case, political enough? My goodness, the joy in life comes from meeting people who are funny or serious in different ways, who are smart on different topics, who are polished in one way and cheerfully unpolished in others, or who are very political and very *not*! So just be you. Give yourself the chance to succeed by being your best self. Maybe you're not expected to be like all the people who came before you; maybe you'll be wanted for being someone brand-new.

If you need reminding of how special you are, get yourself a cheerleader in a friend or family member who'll remind you what you already know: that you were born for this, that you can *do* this. Just do you as truly as you can, and you're paving the path to succeed.

Celebrate the life in loss.

Loss often hits us when we least expect it. And, man, it hits hard. Whether we're grieving a family member, a dear friend, a pet, a companion, or a relationship, desperate to find something positive to hold on to through our pain, perhaps we can find it by celebrating the life rather than the loss.

When I went to my uncle Tommy's wake, it was tough. Tom was my funny uncle. The one who'd shake your hand when you met and ask, "Are you nervous? No? Are you sure? Well, then why are you shaking?" He passed away of a heart attack in the middle of an Irish jig on St. Patrick's Day, and just as we were used to him making us laugh until we cried, it also felt good that day to turn our crying into laughter while sharing stories about his memory. **There is no bright side to a loss itself. But there is light in remembering and celebrating the life that was.**

I had my second miscarriage at seven weeks, and my third at ten weeks, after once again seeing that little heartbeat on the monitor and making plans for a baby room in the coming year. Two days later, I was so overwhelmed by the losses that I drove to the beach in Malibu, sat on the sand beside a rock jetty, and cried loud and strong. I cried for how broken I felt, how confused I was, and how cruel and unfair it seemed that what was so easy for most women was such a struggle for me. But what got me through it was the fact I'd been able to get pregnant at all. I knew not every woman struggling with infertility gets that gift, and even though my three pregnancies weren't successful, I was grateful I'd experienced life inside me at all. I'd loved the cravings I had for peaches and plums, the utter exhaustion I felt all day long, the nausea and twinges within me. There was loss, but I felt lucky that I'd had life.

Sometimes, nothing can describe the depth of grief we feel in losing who we love. The pain of loss even hurts like a physical pain—and because of the stress it puts on your body and emotional intense signals it sends to your brain, it *is* a physical pain.

In fact, a 2011 study by Ethan Kross, PhD, published in the *Proceedings of the National Academy of Sciences* journal, found that the pain of heartbreak activates the same parts of the brain—the secondary somatosensory cortex and the dorsal posterior insula—that true *physical* pain does. The "pain" of loss is real.

But if there is any bright side to it, it's that the grief we feel when we lose someone is in direct correlation to how much love we felt around them in the first place. The life they lived and the joy we gained is what's causing our tears and anguish now. So perhaps it can help for us to think of that as we grieve: It hurts because his or her life *gave* us so much while they were here.

The life we got to share with those we loved—however short or miraculously long—changes us and adds to who we are. And the best gift we can give that person is to be the best part of them and pass on to others what they passed on to us. So if you remember them giving you laughter, find laughter in their spirit. If they helped you feel loved, then be love in their memory. As you carry and work through the loss, celebrate the life. Be the joy.

Follow in Joan's footsteps.

We've all been rejected. For jobs, for loans, by friends, in love. Like the grade school kickball team of life, someone is going to be picked last—and we've all been that someone. But the next time a door shuts on you, open it back up and walk through it; just think like Joan Rivers, who has succeeded in the comedy business—a career *based* on rejection—for more than fifty years.

"You want to hear stupid? Major stupid?" Joan writes in the first line of her first book, *Enter Talking*. "Stand-up comic," she writes, where you walk onto a bare stage totally alone, with everyone judging your personality and whether you're worth their money. "When they do not laugh, that silence is a rejection of you personally, only you," writes Joan. "Not your mother. Not your piano player—if you have one. A thousand people in a room are saying, 'You stink. You're nothing.'" And yet, Joan Rivers stuck it out. When I interviewed Joan for *Angeleno* magazine in Los Angeles, she said that while some people along the way haven't believed in her, she has always believed in herself, and that has made all the difference.

Rejection might make you think, *What do people want from me?* But that's the wrong question. The question to ask is: What do *you* want from you? To do your best, to feel like a good person, to put yourself out there and try? And while you're asking that, ask yourself what you want from *them*. Perhaps you want to be noticed, to be taken seriously, to be appreciated for who you are. And if they don't see that? If they don't choose you? It's their loss. **Someone's rejection of you is *their* problem, not yours. So don't let anyone else's judgment of you change how you feel about yourself.**

Think of the people who've fought back in the face of rejection: Albert Einstein was expelled from school, Walt Disney was once fired by a newspaper editor and J. K. Rowling's first book, *Harry Potter and the Sorcerer's Stone*, was rejected numerous times before Bloomsbury Publishing took it on in 1996 and the series went on to sell hundreds of millions of copies. Following rejection—and perhaps because of it—they've all gone on to far bigger and better things. And think how many people thank the person who dumped them in love for opening them to find the person they were *meant* to be with. Two, four, six, eight, who do they appreciate? If it's not you, good riddance.

If you believe in yourself, don't let other people's lack of faith stop you. When a door closes on you, open it back up and walk right through it. As Joan said onstage in her play *Joan Rivers: A Work in Progress by a Life in Progress*, "I'm seventy-five years old and I tell ya, I haven't peaked. And that is why I'm gonna go out that door. And the door after that. And the door after that. And the door after that. And the door after that. And I invite all of you: Come with me!"

Listen to the woman, will you? She's one who knows. Go through the doors with your head high and your pride intact, for you have so much to offer to the people who are paying attention and are smart enough to appreciate you. Believe in yourself, and their rejection will only make you stronger.

Don't waste worries on the "what-ifs."

My friend Todd recently found himself swimming in a torrent of emotions when he hit a fork in his career. He didn't know if he'd be opening a hair salon in New York or moving to Los Angeles to work with private clients in their homes, and he couldn't take the next step—Did he need an apartment? A car?—in either decision until he heard back from business operators who needed to hear back from their accountants, and so on and so on. Todd kept endlessly running through the "what-ifs" of each possibility until he realized it was getting him nowhere.

"I can handle anything as long as I know what it *is*," Todd finally said. "I can only process what I know." So he let go of the "what-ifs," lived his life, and waited for the answer to land at his feet. Two weeks later, it did, and he's proceeding to open his Bush salon in Manhattan.

Life is sometimes like a game of Twister, when the arrow is still spinning around the color wheel. You can put a foot on yellow and a hand on green if you're told to put it there, but until then, you're in limbo. Like Todd, you can only go full throttle when you know where to head. So until then, **don't waste your energy on what you *don't* know. Instead of worrying about the "what-ifs," take whatever steps you can today. Either take a small first step or put yourself in the hands of life until it tells you what's coming.**

If the choice right now is not up to you, you are only exhausting your logic and tiring your emotions by reviewing the "what-ifs." Because sometimes, there's only so much you can do to *make* things happen. You can make the call, submit your essay, ask for the application, try the technique, put forth the offer, and do your best to get things done. And while it's proactive to review your options, when you reach an end to what you can do—if your "what-ifs" have no answers and you've come back to them more than once—it's time to let it go.

Let the universe lead you where you're supposed to go like the Twister wheel chooses your next color. Just keep your eyes open and look for a sign of which direction to walk. Life just might surprise you. You might learn your "what-if" was pointed in the wrong direction. And "right foot blue" on the Twister board feels more comfortable than you'd think.

Force the run of excitement.

I caught singer Justin Timberlake on an airing of *Ellen* as he was about to turn thirty. When she asked him how he felt about entering his next decade, he said, "I'm excited about my thirties. Yeah, I'm excited about it." Then he paused and smiled. "Well, I don't really have a choice, so I might as well be excited."

I loved that. Sometimes, life hurls you toward something you don't want, but like a forced run in baseball, if you can't control what's happening to you, choose to go forth with excitement.

Maybe you're turning thirty-nine again, or you just qualified for the seniors discount at the movies. Maybe you've been dumped by a partner who's moving their things out on Tuesday and you don't know how to be single all over again. And after a good, healthy cry and the dust of your disappointment has settled, you have a choice about how to face your future. You are *going* to have to take the next step either way, and how you do so is 100 percent up to you. **You may not have a choice about the matter, but you *do* have a choice about your mindset.** So, like the baseball runner who's forced to run home, force yourself to find reasons to like it.

How can you possibly be excited about, say, turning one year older? Well, ask yourself this simple question: *What's one good thing about it?* Here, I'll help you. One year older may bring another gray hair or wrinkle, but those are marks of a life well earned, with nicks and scars and moles and spots that signify every single day you've lived. One year older is one year more of life experience, smarter decision making, and far more confidence. And one year older means you're still living, and that's miraculous. We can all think of a former classmate, coworker, or friend who didn't make it on this earth as far as we have today—and really, what would *they* give for another year, another birthday? Here you are, alive and heading forth into your future.

As bad as a situation feels the moment you find out you're forced into it, find something worth getting excited about.

You're going into this no matter what; you don't have a choice about that. But you *do* have a choice about your mind-set. Look forward to what you'll find at your next base and see how you can score.

Take the tourist's point of view.

I once visited a friend in Miami's South Beach, and since I was flying down from a cold New York winter, the first thing I wanted to do was hit the beach. We laid down our towels and I stepped right into the warm, crystal-clear water.

"This is so amazing," I said. "You must do this every day."

"Actually," he said, "this is the first time I've been to the beach in six months."

Six months! I couldn't believe it! I thought the whole point of Miami *was* the beach. But he lived here; he'd gotten used to it. The same way my friend Dave had come to see London's Abbey Road—now famous for the shot of the Beatles crossing it on the *Abbey Road* album—as just another street by his house.

We do the same in life: We get used to our surroundings, and we simply don't get the same rushes from regular things we do that we did at first. So from time to time, it's good to check in and remember: **The same way travelers seem to appreciate the special things, take the tourist's point of view and see what "wow!" worthy things you have right in front of you.**

Psychologically, it's natural to gain less and less pleasure over time from what's right in front of you. This is known as "habituation," when we get so used to something in our life—our family, phone, pet, partner, or local Chinese take-out spot—and derive less pleasure from it as time goes on. How do you get that pleasure back?

Well, think about how you would show off your town or partner or kitchen to someone who didn't have the same thing. Plan what you'd show off in a superfantabulous double-decker bus tour of that part of your life.

Maybe a tourist looking for a relationship might see how your partner makes goofy jokes at all the commercials, likes doing laundry, and would drop anything to be by your side if you asked. Maybe a tourist who can barely remember what life was like before they had kids might appreciate that you can whisk away for a weekend, get to hog the sheets, practice guitar all night long, and still get butterflies on the way to a first date.

If you're tired of cooking in your same kitchen and driving that same dull route to work, then either add something new to your kitchen and take a different road to the office, or—and this is actually easier—stick with what you've got and look at it from a tourist's point of view. Maybe your kitchen has a dishwasher and a killer espresso machine and a floor that doesn't show dirt. And maybe your drive to work is down a highway that's so steady you can pop in an audiobook and sit back and enjoy the ride in a car with seat warmers that keep you cozy on a chilly day.

Reminders of what to appreciate are all around us. Sometimes it just takes seeing what you have through new eyes. As actress Amy Adams explained to me over breakfast while we talked for *InStyle* magazine, her tourist was her baby daughter. "It's such a great lesson for me," Amy said about how her daughter Aviana approaches the day. "She's never like, 'Oh *God*, I have to eat cereal again and look at the same bouncy seat?' She's always like, 'The bouncy seat?! I remember the bouncy seat! The bouncy seat's awesome!' That," said Amy, "has reminded me about the simple things."

Don't let your life and relationships become the faded old wallpaper you no longer notice. Look—through whatever eyes help you appreciate it—how lucky you are to have what's right in front of you.

Tune into your "real-ometer."

I have to give it to my husband for loving me even when I'm wearing my L.L.Bean men's oversize plaid flannel pajamas. Or, ahem, as he likes to call it, my "suit."

The first cold winter night I put on the pj's after we were married, Gus saw me and said, "Oh, are you going to work?"

"Work?" I asked. "No. Why?"

"Oh," he said, "I thought that's why you're wearing your suit."

I had to look down to notice that with the wide-leg pants

and the big shirt with the buttons and notch collar cut like a men's suit jacket, I did, indeed, look like I was wearing a (terribly work-inappropriate) plaid flannel suit. I laughed, he laughed, and I snuggled up next to him for a long winter's nap.

I still wear the pj's and laugh out loud every time Gus says, "How are things going at the office?" and "Big meeting tonight?" or we decide I need a plaid flannel briefcase to complete the outfit. It's one of the "real-ometers" of our relationship. Gus loves me even when I'm wearing my suit; in fact, he loves me *for* wearing my suit. And we could all use a similar way of judging our relationships—be it with our partners, our friends, or jobs we want. **Your real-ometer measures someone's love for the *real* you. The "you" you want loved most.** And sometimes it goes far past skin-deep.

I learned that when I dated a guy who liked my friends and parents and seemed to have fun when we double dated with my sister and her girlfriend. Three years in, however, I began having doubts about us, but I couldn't put my finger on why. And then, talking about the possibility of getting married, he did it for me.

"Just so you know," he said, "if we get married, I don't want your sister bringing a girl to the wedding. It's not something I believe in and I don't want the spectacle to overshadow our big day."

I was dumbfounded. "So let me get this straight," I said. "You're basically asking me to choose between you and my *sister*."

"I guess," he said.

"Well," I replied, "she wins." I was wiping my hands of him as he dropped me off and I cried with thankfulness for the grace of God or the universe for giving me a sign so clear I couldn't ignore it. Because if someone wasn't going to accept me or my family for exactly who we were, they sure as heck had no place in my life. And the same is true for you: Among friends, at work, and especially in love, it's the real you or nuthin'. If the person you like doesn't call, there are others who will; if a boss doesn't hire you, you'll find jobs you're better off in; and if one friend makes you feel bad about yourself, surround yourself with those who help you feel strong. That's what our real-ometers are: Rather than getting down about those who don't want all of us, a real-ometer lets us see the bright side, the refreshing signs they're not meant to be in our life.

As Tina Fey said in her acceptance speech for the Mark Twain Prize for American Humor: "I met my husband, Jeff, when we were both in Chicago and I had short hair with a perm on top, and I would wear oversize denim shorts overalls. And that is how I know our love is real." Be it perms, patience, or flannel pj's, find yours, too.

Don't salt it before you try it.

I admit it. I put Tabasco sauce in my New England clam chowder before I even taste it because I assume I'll like it better with the kick. And my mom, she salts everything before her first bite because she assumes it won't be flavored to her liking. But as any chef will tell you, these are culinary crimes! How can we possibly know what something's going to taste like before we've taken a spoonful, right? The fair thing to do is give every new dish its own chance to impress us. And the same goes with life—especially our relationships.

Like a palate that develops likes and dislikes due to what we've tasted before, we do the same with people. If we've been hurt or lied to or played or betrayed, this negative programming marks us for life and leads us to look for those signs again in every relationship—whether we're looking for a spouse or searching for a CFO. Our emotional palates are a collection of every feeling we've ever had, every success and every mistake. Because of what we've experienced in the past, our brains—especially the amygdala, two almond-size clusters of neurons in our brain's limbic system—help us make decisions for the future. This is meant to be for our benefit, but it can also inadvertently hold us back. Just as we can't assume a soup needs salt because we tried something similar five years ago, we can't assume we know what a new person will be like because we were hurt by someone similar five years ago. We have to let new people and plates speak for themselves.

Is it helpful to be wary of those who seem similar to people who've hurt you? Absolutely. If you know long-distance relationships or particular types of clients have been tough on you before, then this time around you have to ask the right questions and set boundaries so you don't get pulled down the same road by the same painful patterns all over again. However, **there's being cautious, and there's closing yourself off. Don't let your past make all the decisions for your future. Don't salt your love and relationship experiences before you've even given them a chance.**

Don't assume someone will let you down unless they have. Don't expect they'll screw up unless they do. Don't blanket the people you meet or the person you marry with the issues from those in your past. Don't presuppose a new person is just like everyone else. However your brain has marked you for your past, you must give the people you meet in the present their own chance to show you who they are.

How can you be sure you're giving someone a chance? The next time you fear someone may hurt you, leave you, betray you, or belittle you, ask yourself this: *Do I think this because of something* they've *done, or has this simply happened to me before?* Answer honestly and you may be surprised at what you find. Listen to the red flags and gut reactions from the brain that's been trained to protect you. But don't judge how others will treat you before they've done anything to earn or deserve it. Let down the walls you've put up from your past and give yourself the chance to experience great things with good people today.

Sure, it might need salt—but only *after* you've tasted it. Allowing a dish to speak for itself is how five-star relationships are made.

Hope to it!

My friend Ellen called me after she got home from a dinner party, where her friends had set her up with her potential ideal man.

"I'm so disappointed," Ellen said, explaining that he'd turned out to be weird. "I just . . . I really thought this could be *it*. Why did I get my dumb hopes up again?"

I knew the weariness of hoping so high only to be let down so low. And I also know we struggle with hope because of it. So what's the answer, then? Whatever it is we want in life, should we get our hopes up or lower our expectations? The answer is both; do both at the same time.

That's what hope *is*, after all. Hope is knowing despite what could be bad, you're rooting for a good outcome. If you knew you'd get a positive outcome, you wouldn't have to hope for it, right? Hope only exists when the potential for disappointment is in the room. It's why you have to fight to "keep hope alive," because it *will* fight you back. So expect that you may, somehow, be disappointed, and then hope for a big happy ending. In that way, *in that order*, the formula of hope puts you in a place of strength where you feel confidently prepared for what might come, yet raring for the surprises life may drop in your lap. You fight your flagging energy with a good ol' "hop to it!" and your emotions can buck up in just the same way. Go on, "*hope* to it."

When Ellen goes out at night now, she doesn't expect an instant spark the second she meets a man, so she's not distracted by deep disappointment if she doesn't feel it. Do the same. Having some realistic insight as to what might go wrong is simply like hovering your foot over the break pedal as you approach a curve in the road just in case you have to stop. They call that defensive driving; this is a form of defensive living. Because no matter how good your new job is, you *will* have days you want to stay in bed. And, sorry to say it, but no matter how googly-eyed you feel when you fall in love, you *will* discover a habit that drives you nuts. And as long as you know what could happen, you're ready for the fun part: hoping that this time, for as long as it can, things will all go right.

Great things happen to people all the time, remember. People meet their other halves in love every day. They get their dream jobs and lose the weight and pass the bar exam and get Michelin stars for their restaurants. After my failed pregnancies, I prepared myself emotionally: I knew that my bad experiences probably pointed to a problem, so I steeled my heart that I could be disappointed. But having once seen those plus signs on the pee sticks, I had all the hope in the world I'd see it again.

Hope is a choice. You can *choose* to believe that good things can happen for you. And if you feel you're losing hope, it's up to you to build it back up. Hope isn't a set of keys; you don't reach into the pocket of your down vest and find hope clanging there with sweet relief. You *create* hope within yourself by picturing what could go right. Expect that you might somehow be disappointed, and then hope, in the biggest way you can, to be marvelously surprised. Come on now, hope to it. Life does come through.

When Your
SOCIAL LIFE
Goes a Little Awry...

Dress with your attitude.

When my husband, Gus, was a little boy, he told his mother he needed a costume for a school parade the day after Halloween. A recent immigrant from Argentina, she spoke little English and knew no American traditions, so she followed his lead and got him one he was giddy about.

The morning of the parade, the first-graders settled into the classroom wearing bedroom sheets and blankets in very un-ghostly ways. The parade, it turns out, was a Catholic celebration of All Saints' Day, in honor of each kid's favorite canonized holy being. Girls were swathed in blue like the Virgin Mary; boys wore sheets tied with rope at the waist, holding fake shepherd staffs like St. Joseph. And Gus? He marched in dressed as *Star Wars*'s Chewbacca. His teachers still let him walk in his fuzzy suit that day, but the families attending the All Saints' Day parade had never had such a good laugh.

We've all had a moment like that in spirit. We're overdressed or underdressed. We're in the wrong place for the wrong event. We've shown up with the wrong materials and the wrong questions and can't see how to make it right. What does it make us want to do? Crawl under a rock and hide until the sun sets. What do I suggest we do instead? Embrace the awkwardness and change what you look like from the inside out.

That's because we appear on the outside how we feel on the inside. Dressing isn't as much about the fabric draped on your body as how you carry it. It's why some women can wear discount clothes that seem couture, and some men can make skateboard sneakers look rad with a business suit. **It's not the fabric on your back but the attitude underneath it that makes all the difference.** It's why I've dressed up for a fancy party wearing high heels I wish would turn into slippers past midnight, and envied the girl in jeans and flats who somehow looks more comfortable than me. And why a proud Gus was no longer embarrassed about his costume when a saintly classmate said, "I wish I was wearing my Han Solo costume."

If you find yourself uncomfortable in how you look or where you are, change your attitude outfit: Throw your shoulders back, stand up tall, lift your chin, and smile. Say to yourself, "I'm glad I'm wearing/doing/reading/carrying this, and soon, they'll all wish they were, too." The truth is, no one's thinking too hard about what you're wearing (they're too busy thinking about themselves), but once you're wearing your confidence, others will envy it. Luckily, dressing with your attitude can be done in every size, in every season.

"Oh, this old thing?" you can say. "I was feeling it, so I just threw it on."

Seek out a "smiler."

Jokes may make us smile, but smiling is no joke. So when you feel like nothing in the world can make you smile, your best offense may be to do just that. Smile for fifteen seconds, a grin big enough to engage your cheeks and wrinkle your crow's-feet like you do in a genuine smile. Because the sheer act of smiling—even if you're forcing it—creates changes in our autonomic nervous system, sends dopamine through our brains, and produces feelings of happiness.

But what if you can't force it? What if—even knowing that smiling will help—you can't seem to make yourself do it? Then reach out for unconscious help from someone else. Seek out a smiler.

Here's why: The frontal lobe of the brain contains bundles of neurons known as "mirror neurons" that respond to what other people are expressing and feeling. If you've ever noticed your forehead scrunching in empathy while someone on a talk show tells their sad story, or felt the pain of a NASCAR driver climbing out of a crushed car, you've experienced the effects of your mirror neurons. They create an emotional feedback loop, known as "empathic resonance," that makes you able to "catch" someone else's mood. It's as if your brain seeing someone *else* do something is the same as doing it yourself. And studies have shown it works with smiling: **By seeing someone else smile, you're able to "catch" their mood by smiling and feeling happier yourself.**

Take it from researchers in a 2002 study at Sweden's Uppsala University. They showed participants photos of smiling, frowning, and expressionless faces and instructed them to make similar and opposite faces in return. As they were hooked up to equipment that measured electrical signals in their faces, Dr. Ulf Dimberg and his team were able to measure their facial reactions, and this is the cool part: They found that when participants viewed a smiling face, it was very difficult for them to follow the direction to frown, and vice versa. That, my friends, are those mirror neurons at work. When you see a smiling face, it's hard as heck not to smile back.

So seek out a smiler and borrow their mood—then turn around and pass it on.

Give a gratitude shout-out.

My friend Jackie was going through a hard time in both her career and her dating life. And while none of her life puzzle pieces were fitting together, she noticed that while she had some down spots every day, one or two people would always say or do something that made her feel better.

"I call them my angels," she told me during a lunch break from work. For even though she's not religious, she felt like people were being sent to support her when she really needed it. One day, her boss gave her some well-needed praise for a job she'd done. Another day, a friend passed along a compliment a cute guy said about her. And one day, it was a stranger who asked where she got her cute shoes.

"Every night, before I go to bed," said Jackie, "I write down who my angel was, to remind me to be grateful for what I have." And when, a few months later after a catch-up phone call, Jackie emailed to say she was putting me down as her angel that day, tears welled up in my eyes. I don't know what I'd said on the telephone, but it made me want to thank someone who'd helped *me* have a better day, too. Because even when your day is feeling down, **keep your eyes open for people who shift it in some small way—with a kind word, a warm hug, or a friendly glance. Give those people a shout-out.**

And if you're not up for making a list of angels every day, consider doing it once a year, as *My Last Wishes* author Joy Meredith does in a tradition she calls her "Thanksgiving List." First, Joy makes a list of all the people in her life she's grateful for, then, on Thanksgiving morning, she calls and tells each friend specifically why. "On the morning of Thanksgiving," says Joy, "I wake up early, make two Pepperidge Farm cherry turnovers, and begin my calls around nine-ish. Working off my notes, I take a moment to get present with my gratitude and then I call my friend Ann—the list is alphabetical—and begin the thanking. It is designed to be a quick call; there are no pleasantries or small talk. It starts: "Are you ready? Okay, Ann, this is why I am thankful for you this year . . ." She'll thank one friend for letting her carve pumpkins with her kids, making her feel so included in the kids' lives; she'll thank another for treating her to a nice lunch back in April and being the first to call when she landed a new job.

Of course it makes friends feel good, but there's just as much in it for you. "There is no better way to inventory your life and successes than to see who helped you along the way," Joy explains. "Some say it is a generous thing to do, but really it is all about me listing how great my life is and who I've come to love along the way. It really, truly is the best gift I give *myself* all year."

In a life so often spent rushing to work or grumbling our way up the drugstore line with a pack of paper towels in our arms, it changes us for the better to tune into the small moments of positivity from people we're grateful for—and ideally, we tell them just that. Another friend of mine has a tradition that over birthday dinners for her friends, everyone at the table takes a turn sharing a meaningful story or a quality they've appreciated about the birthday honoree. Yeah, it makes the guest of honor blush a bit, but what better way to build up someone you love than by reminding him or her what makes you stick around.

Go on, make your own Thanksgiving List. Write down

your angels. Tell your loved ones why you're celebrating. Give 'em all a gratitude shout-out. And keep spreading the actions of an angel in your everyday life because, as we've experienced for ourselves, sometimes that's just what a person really needs.

Gaffe in all your glory!

A few years ago, I was in a department store dressing room trying on a dress that was supposed to flow over and under the arms and around my back like a runway piece. But when I tried to wiggle into it, somewhere between sticking my arms up and pulling the dress down . . . it got stuck. Like, actually stuck.

I couldn't bend my elbows to pull it farther up or down, and with the fabric of the bodice covering my face, I couldn't see into the mirror to figure out what the heck I was doing wrong. I spent five minutes wiggling around like Houdini in a strait-jacket, which got me nothing but tired and unnecessarily pan-icked. *Oh my God,* I started thinking. *What if I can't get out of this? What if I suffocate and die?* What can I say, terror comes easily when your ready-to-wear attacks. I needed some of that dressing room assistance.

"Uh, hello?" I asked feebly through the cotton/silk blend in front of my face. "Is anyone in here?"

"Yes?" I heard a woman answer.

"I, um, sort of need help?" I whimpered. "I'm kind of . . . stuck."

We played a little dressing room Marco Polo until she found me. But with my arms stuck at my ears in "tree pose" inside the fabric, I realized, *I can't unlock the door.* The woman got an employee to open it and the two of them untangled me from the fabric—which then left me, of course, standing naked in nothing but the ugly baggy undies I wear when I *don't* plan on strangers seeing me naked. Standing there bare, blushing and embarrassed, I said something like, "Wow, styles today," and got out fast.

Embarrassing gaffes are tough. But they happen all the time. You're stuck in a stall with no toilet paper. The bathroom door doesn't lock. Or the bathroom locks *so* well you have to knock from the inside to get back out. Or the restaurant's glass door won't open when you pull it, and all the patrons inside get to watch you struggle before you see it says "Push." Or maybe your date (like mine once did) mistakes the wasabi for a split pea mash and eats a tablespoon of it in one nasal-burning gulp and makes a scene begging for water to wash it down.

But the truth is, after you've done something embarrassing, you've actually gained two very useful things. One, you're more likable. A 1966 study by psychologist Elliot Aronson and his colleagues Willerman and Floyd about the "pratfall effect" found goofs like this can actually increase your attractiveness to others. **Remember this: When you make a big misstep, you simply seem more human and people are more apt to warm up to you because you're more of a possible friend than a potential threat.**

The other bonus to embarrassing gaffes: Hilariously uncomfortable moments are what life is all about! Yes, we feel out of our element. But guess what? An uncomfortable moment is a sign we're alive. If you've never felt like you're on unfamiliar ground, you may be stuck *inside* your element and have gotten *too* comfortable. Routine, of course, can be lovely; I think there's great happiness to be found in the same hot cup of tea every day. But it's also healthy for us to put ourselves in places that challenge us, and to persevere through it until you land safely back on familiar turf. Breaking new ground can be embarrassing, but it's also *living*. And when the blush fades, you may at least have a story that leads to a lifetime of laughs you can share with your friends. And please, oh please, share them with me.

Ask, WWMRMD?

Sometimes, when you find yourself about to lose it, you yourself may not be the best judge of what you yourself should do. And in those cases, I suggest following the lead of those who might ask WWJD: What Would Jesus Do? Asking what Jesus would do leads some people in the right direction, and you can do the same for yourself. Choose a role model and ask what they'd do. *WWMRMD*: What Would My Role Model Do?

Changing perspectives gets you out of the box you're in and looking at it from another angle. Maybe your role model is a family member whose logic never fails or a friend you've always respected. Or maybe it's a quirky iconic character you've seen on TV: What would McNulty from *The Wire* do? Carrie Bradshaw from *Sex and the City*? Columbo? By coming at it from people who might approach your situation differently, you create more options about what might be best. Because in the heat or struggle of a moment, **by focusing on a person you respect, you'll make respectable decisions as the person you are.**

In Woody Allen's 1972 film *Play It Again, Sam*, anytime Allen's character found himself floundering in a dating situation, tough guy actor Humphrey Bogart appeared as a ghost and told him, well, what Humphrey Bogart would do. In the book *The Game*, author Neil Strauss talks about interviewing Tom Cruise for *Rolling Stone* and being awed by the actor's alpha male ability to control the room; when Strauss later found his buttons pushed by an annoying acquaintance, he thought, *What would Tom Cruise do?* and handled the situation flawlessly. It's a great tool when you need it.

If you find yourself wanting to slam down the phone on a needy client, yell at a customer service rep, sheepishly turn away from a party you're about to walk into alone, or you're panicked before a pitch meeting, ask yourself: *What would _____ do?*

For me, anytime I appear on TV, I picture my friend Suze, a regular on the small screen, sitting down with me before my first television appearance. She drew a big happy face on a piece of white paper with a Sharpie, then held it up in front of the camera.

"That's your audience," she told me, beaming as big as the happy face. "They're your friends!"

Now, if I want to lose my lunch as we're about to go live, I think of her: *What would Suze do?* Well, she'd smile and tell her friends all the fun stuff she knows. In a tough moment, do the same. Turn to your role models. When you ask WWM-RMD, you'll find yourself acting and feeling just like them.

Be friendly first.

Christoph Brown had the rough shift at a Los Angeles coffee shop: When he awoke at five a.m. to open the store, he was the first to greet grumbling customers shuffling in for a cup of nicer personality. "My cup of coffee started my customers' day, and I knew how I acted with them would affect how their whole day went from there," says Brown. "So I'd be friendly to set the mood of the morning. For the grouchiest customers, I would see if I could change their energy with a smile, and it worked."

When, a few months later, a customer left behind a pocket-size Etch A Sketch, Christoph sketched someone's face in minutes and propped it up by the register. So many customers reacted positively that he bought himself a few more small toys to play around with, and five years later, he's now running his own entertainment business, sketching for private and public events as the Amazing Etch Man. And it all began by being the friendly one first. He not only made people smile those mornings in the coffee shop, he's made a career out of it.

The lesson is a good one. When we first interact with someone, we may wait for that person to be positive first, so we can react and respond to their approach. But why wait for someone else to set the mood when we have the power to do it ourselves—and make it 100 percent positive? Like Christoph, **you can change the dynamic of a moment or a day by choosing to be the *first* one to be friendly.** Take the initiative. Introduce yourself first with a big smile. Be the first one to offer to grab them a drink. Be the first one to notice someone's new haircut, beautiful briefcase, or killer shoes. Be the first one to ask how their day's been and what they're looking forward to tomorrow. It works whether you're on a date, in a business meeting, at a family event, or approaching a customer service representative about a return. You can tilt the experience to a positive one by leading it there yourself. This also works in your own living room. Want the mood in your home with your partner to be a brighter, warmer one? Take it there first with consideration, a soft kiss, or a shoulder rub. By setting a mood of warm and friendly first, you'll give your other half a chance to do the same.

It really is that simple. Be friendly first and you create a space and an energy in which others can respond in kind—literally. It can enhance your relationships, help build new ones, and like a smile that comes with a cup of coffee, nudge your everyday interactions toward positive outcomes. Give people opportunities to be their best, and they just might surprise you.

Listen for the gems.

I was standing at a bus stop in Washington, DC, the day I learned how to listen. I was reading a book when an old man in his eighties inched up beside me and launched into an "I remember when" story of how the street we were on used to be a dirt logging road when he was in the navy. I "mmm"-ed and "uh-huh"-ed on cue.

"It took me across the world once," said the old man. "We were supposed to go to Italy, my wife and I. I'd always promised I'd take her around the world, but we'd never been. So when our flight was delayed, I said we could get there by going around the world the *other* way!"

His rambling words began to entice me with that one, and his eyes, lit by the fire of his memories, grew brighter as he passed the story through his tingling senses and into mine.

"We went to the darndest countries," he said, "even though we didn't have much money—heck, *we* didn't know we'd be going around the world! And you know how we got along?" he said. "By talking to people, you know?" I was starting to.

"In one place," he said, "we were on this bus and I asked a man, 'Sir, could you tell me how to say three things?' And do you know what three things I asked him?" I shook my head. "I asked him 'bread,' 'cheese,' and 'wine.' And when we got into town, we found a little store with a little counter, and I handed him the piece of paper with those three words written on it—bread, cheese, and wine—and the man, he called over a boy and sent him across the street. Then he took a loaf of fresh bread from a shelf and comes back with some cheese. Well, then the boy runs in and do you know what he's holding? A bottle o' wine!"

The bus pulled to the curb to pick us up and as I let him step on ahead of me, I began to memorize this man. He turned from the steps and said, "Just one more story on the bus, and then I'll leave you alone." We sat next to each other, and he told me how his wife had died, and how he remarried a woman with seven wonderful children.

"But it was hard," he said, "because I loved my first wife so much . . ."

There I sat, soaking in all I could for the future, and there he sat, wringing out what he could from the life he'd lived. "My wife," he said, "the one I just told you about? She died a few months ago. It's hard being alone again, you know?"

I did know. I knew that people needed to talk to people—in foreign countries or at local bus stops—in order to survive. The man stood up as the bus slowed to a stop, leaned over, and shook my hand. "Well, okay, then," he said. As he walked toward the front of the bus, I wanted to get off and follow him, tell him that he wasn't wasting his time on me, that I really *was* listening. That it changed me. Sure, I sometimes still plug my ears with headphones and bury my face in a book to keep strangers in public from talking to me. But sometimes, I don't.

Years later, in fact, I was the one who stopped to talk to another older gentleman who was waiting for a Jitney bus heading out of Manhattan. He was dressed nicely, banging a metal fence with a pair of drumsticks. I was so intrigued that on my way home from work, I stopped and talked to him about detective novels for half an hour. Then I asked him about the drumsticks.

"I was just at a benefit for my son's foundation," he said. "Maybe you've heard of him. Harry Chapin?" Wow. Harry Chapin, who famously sang "Cat's in the Cradle," about sons and dads—this was Harry's *dad*, Jim Chapin, a musician in his own right.

The point is, we all have times we don't feel like talking. We want to keep to ourselves on the subway platform, or waiting room, or train. And when a stranger interrupts our peace, we don't want to hear it. **But there's a gem hidden in every conversation: Either you get a gift of hearing it or you *give* a gift by listening.**

There are gems in every conversation. Listen and you shall give and receive.

Elevate the throwaways.

What's one of the first exchanges they teach you when you're learning a new language? No, the one right after "Where's the toilet?" Okay, and the one *after* "One more beer, please." Yes, *that* one. The one that goes like this:

"Hi, how are you?"

"I'm fine. How are you?"

In every language, in every culture, we use that phrase nearly every day. We use it so much it's become a rote exchange, a total throwaway. But we waste precious opportunities to connect with people when we blindly follow life's pre-scripted dialogue. **Think what could happen if you embraced those rote moments as real ones. Connect more with the people you interact with during the day by elevating the throwaways.**

Life's throwaways can be elevated into astonishing things, remember. You can turn what you'd toss out in your kitchen into fresh compost that grows twice as many tomatoes, or, like Malawi resident William Kamkwamba, coauthor of his story *The Boy Who Harnessed the Wind*, you can turn scrap metal and tractor parts into a working windmill that powers lightbulbs in the family home. And throwaway words—the ones you'd usually toss out—can be just as powerful when you embrace them.

The next time someone asks how you are, answer honestly. "I'm doing pretty well, actually." Or "All things considered, pretty darn awesome." And if things aren't going well, try honesty with a positive twist—because elevating your throwaways into one gnarly grouch-fest isn't going to make you feel better. Instead try, "I've had better days. I'm looking forward to a fresh start tomorrow." Or, "It's not great. Tell me something good about yours!"

And you don't just have to elevate your "hellos." You can raise the bar on all sorts of quick exchanges. Turn "thanks" at the checkout line into, "Thanks for doing that so quickly," or

"Thank you very much. Now I can't wait to go home and eat all this!" Turn "Excuse me" in a crowd into, "Sorry, hate to squeeze past you like this." Or turn what normally might be a quick nod of the head or no acknowledgment at all—with neighbors you don't know, the person you pass in the office building lobby—into a warm hello to change how you both feel in two seconds flat.

And in your other communications, reach a higher level with the smallest of words. Behold, for example, the power of "so," says Larry Rosen, PhD, psychology professor at California State University and author of *iDisorder*. That small word can do wonders to your relationships at work and in life. "It's 'I'm happy to meet you' versus 'I'm *so* happy to meet you,'" Rosen told me. "And 'I appreciate what you did for me' versus 'I *so* appreciate what you did for me.' The word 'so' is free, but it elevates what seems to be a throwaway to a level of more importance and a deeper interaction."

Elevate your throwaways like Kamkwamba powered lightbulbs and you, too, can brighten an average day.

. . . .

Gift someone their own name.

. . . .

I was walking out of a photo shoot when I saw one last person I wanted to bid good-bye, so I popped my head into her office.

"Bye, Lisa!" I said. "So great meeting you."

She nodded back slowly with a weird look on her face.

149

Sheesh, what's up with her? I thought. Two hours later, while retrieving a phone number on the call sheet, I found out what was up with her: Lisa's name was Kathy.

This happens a lot: We're introduced to a man at a party and eleven seconds later have no idea what his name is, or we've met a woman six times and as she approaches with open arms, we wonder, *How the heck do I* still *not know her name?* And what we often do when our memory deals us an empty "My Name Is" badge is dance around it, saying things like, "Oh, *you* . . . !" while desperately seeking someone to swoop in and clear it up. The next time you don't know someone's name, I suggest this instead: Ask for the name again so you can give them the gift of using it.

Names are like little presents. Like a gift someone buys "just for you," a name is the same thing: It highlights the essence of what makes you unique from the person standing next to you. The second someone uses your name, they're expressing that they're not talking to everyone, they're talking to you—to special, unique you. My cat doesn't know a single word of the English language no matter how many times I say "food" and "jump" and "fetch." But when I say, "Guinness," she turns her head, leaps on my lap, and purrs. I think we humans purr inside the very same way.

In fact, a 2007 study by Dennis P. Carmody and Michael Lewis found that entirely different sections of the brain are activated when hearing one's own name compared to others. Neurally and emotionally, we like to hear ourselves reflected back to us, in word and in name. So give others the gift—even if it means stepping up and asking them again. It's not an insult to forget someone's name, but it *is* an insult to dodge them because you have. The way I see it, **it's far better to ask someone's name and use it than dance around the awkwardness of not knowing. Give others the small gift of their name whenever you can.**

How do you do it? Well, you *decide* to. I got so tired of saying, "Oh, I'm so bad with names," I tried to be good with them. And I've succeeded, for the most part, by focusing solely on the person I'm meeting for a few solid moments and using that memory gold standard of repetition. And if I forget it a few minutes later—or, yeah, a few seconds later—I'll admit it. "I'm sorry," I might say. "I completely spaced when you told me your name. What is it again?" Because that's what I hope someone would do for me.

A rose may smell as sweet by any other name, but if it had ears, I think the little buddy would bloom with pride if you called it by the right one.

Climb into the boat of great company.

It's hard being the only one. The only single person at the wedding. The only one wide-awake at three a.m. The only one hitting a rocky patch in your relationship. The only one pissed off at the lady who cut the line at the supermarket. But you're not.

We're not. **We're in this stuff together, all of us. And sometimes, just knowing there's a world of people in the same boat, feeling just as you are right now, is enough to help you through it.**

Climbing into that boat is how I overcame having panic attacks years ago. Because what I hadn't realized was that keeping the secret of my attacks—you know, the "While you guys were laughing at the movie and gnawing on Twizzlers, I thought I was having a heart attack and almost jumped up and yelled for an ambulance"—was only making them worse. The minute I started talking about it, others came clean, too. And once we started sharing the places we'd been blindsided—at brunch, in church, in the middle of a meeting at work—we not only felt better, we started laughing about it. There we were, intelligent adults, falling for the monsters under the bed. And the harder we laughed, the more we stripped the power from the panic. We no longer felt alone, and we all suffered from them less. In solidarity comes strength. Whatever you're going through, there are others in that boat.

Remember that the next time you feel like the odd one out: You're not the only one who feels like you're swimming in debt. You're not the only one who's lonely. You're not the only one feeling lost about your career, or wishing people in the movie theater would stop texting. You're *not* the only one. Take comfort in that.

When I got some genetic testing to find a reason for my failed pregnancies, I was diagnosed with a chromosomal condition that makes it less likely I'll have a healthy pregnancy.

I was crushed at the news and sat stunned in the car the whole ride home from the doctor's office. But in searching for strength, I found endless support in reading stories of other couples diagnosed with the same disorder. Even though I didn't contact any of them, I felt like we were in it together. I ravenously read and related to their accounts and, noting their advice, felt better than ever about taking our next step in treatment to start the family we wanted to have. I was in great company, I wasn't alone. And with every "Why me?" moment, spouting tears at the sight of a baby or at the news of another pregnant friend, I was reminded it's really a "Why us?" This infertility thing that's going around? I'm not the only one; we're not alone.

Whatever the rough waters in your life, there are others going through the same difficulties on other coasts and in other countries. Let them support you in spirit. In big problems and in small, we are all in this together. Climb in the boat and you'll see.

Set your own sound track.

My cousin Christopher celebrated his bachelor party before his wedding by renting a boat for a week with his brother and a few friends in Texas. As they pulled into dock their first night, Christopher hopped out to guide the boat into the slip, but misjudged where the front of the boat was. The vessel, coming in fast, pinned his leg between the boat and a rock, and sliced his calf open, separating his muscle from his bone. He was taken by helicopter to a nearby hospital, far from his Baltimore home, and as he lay in bed in the trauma unit in San Antonio, he not only kept his spirits high, he made jokes. Why?

"The accident was bad enough in and of itself because of the pain, the timing, and my fear of what would happen to my leg," Christopher told me, "that there was no reason to scare others or focus on the crappiness of the situation, which would only make it worse. So I started having fun with the doctors and was happy when talking to friends and family, because I found that by getting *other* people to relax and have more fun around me, it made the situation easier for me to handle." Just like setting the mood of a moment with a musical sound track, we have the power to set the tone of our experiences: **Don't let life choose a tone of fear or uncertainty for you; set your own sound track for life, and the calm or happiness will come right back to you.**

For three weeks, anytime someone asked Chris how he was doing, he answered, "I'm better today than I was yesterday but not as good as I'll be tomorrow." As Christopher puts it, "I'm no psychologist, but that was probably more beneficial for me to say than it was for others to hear. But it calmed people down. I really found that by being upbeat, others were, too, which in turn made me feel a bit better about the whole thing."

On a sunny Saturday in Baltimore three weeks later, Christopher hobbled up the church aisle on a cane at his wedding with a grin on his face, and we danced and ate and laughed our way through the great celebration he still got to have.

You can do this anytime you find yourself in a situation where the tone isn't what you wish for it to be. Maybe you make a sleepy classroom of kids stand up and do jumping jacks. Maybe you get your downbeat friends at dinner to take turns telling their "worst date" stories to lighten the mood. Maybe you assure your frowny-faced family that you're still able to enjoy other aspects of life as you slog through your health struggle. Or maybe you tell your friends you're doing okay after a breakup in love.

When actress Sandra Bullock stood onstage to accept an MTV Generation Award a few months after separating from her cheating husband, she put the tense room at ease by saying, "Can we please go back to normal? Because therapy is really expensive," she joked. "Go back to making fun of me, I don't care. It's time to get back to normal." She knew how to set the tone, and others followed.

Start your own cycle of calm or happiness or generosity or fun by setting your own sound track for life.

....

Make the worst the best.

....

A few days before our tax appointment this year, my husband and I were already worn out, having spent the week organizing receipts and adding up bills.

"This," said Gus, "is absolutely, by far, the worst day of the year."

I agreed. But I wished I didn't have to.

"You know what?" I said. "Maybe we should start trying to turn the *worst* day of the year into the absolute *best*." Then we created one we would look forward to.

Our appointment was just before lunch, so right afterward, we headed to a fab little French restaurant and ordered *moules frites* and two glasses of wine—the grown-up's edition of a postgame ice-cream cone. After lunch, we rode our bikes to the beach and put our feet in the sand, then went home and snuggled into bed for an afternoon nap. By the end of the day—after ordering in spicy eggplant and egg rolls from our favorite Chinese place—we were grinning over what a perfect day we'd had, and were already brainstorming about what we'll do after next year's tax appointment to make it even better (the word "go-kart" has been tossed around). From now on, instead of dreading our "worst" day of the year, we'll be looking forward to our best.

There are endless ways to turn the worst events, experiences, or appointments into the best, the same ways singers turn their breakups into their biggest hit songs: Turn the broken eggs you wanted to poach into the best frittata. Make a meeting you really don't want to attend a prerequisite to getting the best massage. A boring speech you wouldn't normally sit through can become a bingo game. And you can always turn a list of dreaded to-dos into a fun-filled day with a friend: Meet for a hearty breakfast, then hit all of your stops—to get bolts at the hardware store, drop off your broken lamp at the lighting shop, and fix the ring that needs resizing at a jewelry place. Celebrate the joy of getting it done with a cocktail, a dessert, or a pedicure with the works.

Stop dreading the worst of what life has to offer by finding a way to make it the best. The lame things in life have nuthin' on an imagination of the best you can be.

Why can't "someday" be now?

Before I met Gus, I made a dream board of what I wanted my life to look like, with photos of cute babies, lobster lunches, palm trees, and vacations. When he saw the picture I'd posted of Machu Picchu, he said, "I want to go there, too."

"Maybe we will someday," I said.

Three years later, after we got married, we were in my office where my dream board is still posted on the wall above my printer.

"I wonder when we'll go to Machu Picchu," I said.

"I don't know," he answered. "Someday."

"You know what?" I said. "Why can't someday be now?" After all, we thought we'd have kids by now, but because of our bad luck with my health issues, it was still just the two of us. *Maybe,* I thought, *we should be making the most of our unintended freedom.* Maybe life was telling us the window was now.

"I think we should do it," I said. "I think we should go to Machu Picchu."

"Okay," Gus replied. And that was that.

Six months later, just after the sun rose, we stepped onto the misty grasses of the ancient site of Machu Picchu to the sound of chirping birds and the Urubamba River rushing at the base of the mountain. "I can't believe we're actually here," we said, after twelve days of travel through Argentina and into Peru. We were moved by the place and proud of ourselves for doing it. And we've continued to do our somedays now more than ever. Before we took the next big step in our quest to start a family by getting science—and seven-inch needles— involved, we went to Japan, where we walked the vibrant streets of Tokyo and said prayers for our future family at the temples in Kyoto. And to celebrate my recent birthday, we went all out with a road trip through the jungles and beaches of Costa Rica. We're taking our somedays while we have them. Because "someday" will never happen unless you let it.

Today, after all, was *one* day's "someday." When you said you wanted to do something, visit something, try something, or start something "someday," that day could have been today. **If there are things you wish you could start, trips you wish you could take, places you wish you could see "someday," why can't someday be now?**

When I was little, my nana had a magnet on her fridge—a circular button with four capital letters on it: TUIT. "I always said I would do things when I got around to it," my nana explained, "so someone gave me a round 'tuit.' Now I have no excuses." I didn't get it as a kid, but now I understand it more than ever. Our lives are just so full of, well, life. We can't plan ahead for next week, let alone slot the "someday." Or we think it'll be too complicated with the kids or the dogs or the planning. Or we're so sure we want to do that "someday" thing with someone special that we put it off until that day comes. But here's the thing: If you never schedule it, someday may never happen. And while "someday, somewhere, somehow" sounds wistful when Barbra Streisand sings it, in our lives, it's just a shame. You deserve to live your dreams. Not someday, *now*.

So here's what I suggest: Choose a big item on your "someday" list—be it a vacation trip, an alteration to your home, or getting certified in scuba—then pick a day on your calendar that looks like "someday" to you. That first week of March, maybe? The end of May? Or maybe a year from now, to celebrate the anniversary of your pluckiness.

Next, make a list of what needs to happen—be it calling contractors for estimates, researching hotels, or bringing lunch to work for four months to cover the cost. Once you have it on the calendar and a plan to move forward, it's not a someday anymore. It's March fourth. Or May thirtieth. Or October tenth. Which means you won't waste the days you have today dreaming of a someday instead of living it. Life is short. And some experiences will be far better now than later—while your hips and energy are still up to the task.

Take it from my great-uncle Bill Dietrich, who was eighty-six when he gave me some life advice more than a decade ago. "Eat all the spices you can," he said. "When I was younger, I could eat anything. But now, when I go out to a restaurant, I can't eat any spices; it bothers me later on. And I miss a big steak. A good sirloin steak. It's too much work trying to chew on that." He passed away a few years ago, and I think of him when I order good steaks and spicy food. Don't waste life dreaming. Live it doing. Unlike my nana, I know you don't need your own TUIT. Because you can get around to it—*soon*-day if you can.

When
FAMILY AND FRIENDS
Are Stressing You Out . . .

See "help" is not a
four-letter word.

I was thirty when I finally learned that asking for help is not a sign of weakness.

I needed an air conditioner one sweltering summer day in New York City. Single at the time and stubborn that I could do it on my own, I headed to the Kmart on Astor Place. Hauling my new air conditioner into the cart and rolling it to the register was no big deal; but when I walked outside, I had to lug the 140-pound box up thirty steps to street level to get it into a taxi. Still, I thought, *I got this*. I lifted the box up slowly, step by step, sweat bead by sweat bead. Yeah, this was going to take a while.

About eight steps up, a guy on the street called down to me. "You need some help?" he asked.

"No, that's okay," I grunted. "I got it."

He raced down anyway, grabbed the air conditioner box from me, and walked it up the steps. "You need help getting it into a cab?" he asked.

"I got it," I said. "I'm sure I can . . . I mean, I should be fine."

He stepped into the street anyway, hailed me a cab, knocked on the trunk, and lifted the box in for me. My eyes began watering with gratefulness, for, without him, I *so* would not have "got it."

"All good?" he said.

"All good," I said, nearly whimpering. I wanted to hug him. Instead, I stammered out a little "thank you," climbed into the cab, and sobbed. I sobbed because I was so grateful for the kindness of a stranger to offer to help me, and I sobbed because I couldn't believe it had been so hard for me to *let* him. When the taxi pulled up in front of my place, I asked the driver for helping carrying the box four flights up my walk-up.

Of course then I spent the next two days kicking things and cursing as I installed the air conditioner in my window *without* asking for help. Did it feel good to get it in on my own? Yes. Would I have felt just as good doing it in a quarter of the time with someone at my side? Probably. But I'm working on remembering that help is not a four-letter word.

It's not a flaw if we're overwhelmed and admit it. In fact, I don't know about you, but I've always seen people who've asked me for help—or hired others to help them—as strong, bold, together. I envy how wise they are to know they're tapped out and how fearless they are to fix it. **Asking for help is a sign of strength. It says you know your capabilities and your limits, and you could simply use a hand to get things done.**

Ask for help cleaning, carrying, proofreading, cooking, babysitting, and if you need a good word put in for you about a job. And when someone offers to bring you soup when you're sick or pick up a colander for you when they're at IKEA, take them up on it! This is what family and friends are for, to pick up some slack when we need it. You'll feel better having some of the burden lifted, and it will make your family and friends—or maybe even a complete stranger—feel great in helping you, too.

Don't wait until a weight on your shoulders is crushing you and you're no good for anyone. Let your family and friends help you be the person they love most—which is probably the you that's *not* crying on the side of a road trying to haul a heavy air conditioner home alone. To be your best you, sometimes you don't "got it." Sometimes you'll need a hand. Let people give you one.

Give an unconditional gift.

Ralph Waldo Emerson wrote in his classic essay "Gifts" that "the only gift is a portion of thyself." But sometimes, it can feel as if that's *all* you're giving, right? Small chunks of your time, your effort, and your energy without getting equal parts in return. And the moment we feel taken advantage of by friends, in love, at work, or by family, we become so focused on the checks and balances that we start keeping score to make sure we *get* what's owed to us: Since we're the ones who bought the wine for dinner, filled up the gas tank, and watched a friend's kids in an emergency the last six times, where's the payback?

The problem is, that even-steven mentality is, at heart, pessimistic. It assumes that if you continue to work or give or say yes, you'll only end up screwed. Certainly, in some instances of toxic relationships, it's healthy to step back and say no. But other times, you may benefit more from the optimistic approach to giving: *Don't* think about what you'll get in return and tune into how good it feels to brighten someone else's day. **Give an unconditional gift, without wanting or expecting a thing in return.**

My friend Beth Greenwald is exceptional at this—as humble as she is when I tell her so. When we met a couple from Europe celebrating their retirement at happy hour, Beth bought them their final round. When she pulled up to the take-out window at Del Taco and overheard the employee finding out she had to work an extra hour, Beth gave her a twenty for a few tacos, said, "The change is for you," and sped off before the girl could react. And then there was the night she went to Benihana for a dose of fried rice and heard the young couple next to her had just gotten engaged. After Beth saw the ring—with a setting bigger than the diamond—and heard them debating if they should spring for the extra shrimp, she and her friend both paid for their meal. "I wasn't going to let them stress out over the money they were spending to celebrate!" Beth said. The bride-to-be teared up with gratefulness (and yes, they got the extra shrimp). Beth also sponsors a child in Namibia, offers regular loans to Kiva.org, and, in lieu of gifts for her birthday, asks friends to help fund a classroom in need through DonorsChoose.org.

"What makes you do all these things?" I finally asked, seeing as how these random acts of giving so rarely occur to me.

"What do you mean?" she said. "Why wouldn't I?"

And there you go. Why wouldn't we? Giving feels good. Especially when we're not looking to get something from it.

Unconditional giving doesn't require money, either. It can mean just as much and sometimes more to offer your time, your advice, or your ear. Think about a friend who needs a shoulder to lean on, a ride to the mechanic, an invitation to a fun night out, or a compliment, and offer it. Think about an acquaintance either celebrating or mourning an occasion—a birthday, a wedding anniversary, the anniversary of a parent's death—and send a kind note of support. Think about a neighbor who could use a babysitter, an extra hand to make appetizers for a holiday fete, or a second opinion on their résumé, and provide it. Think about an organization that could use your hands or a few nonperishables and donate what you can.

When you give without expecting a single thing in return, you can experience the joy of selflessness, which can be enough to turn off the temptation to tally what you are or aren't getting back. When you "give a portion of thyself" this freely, you won't even miss it. And you'll feel happier about letting it go.

··

Make the most of your middle.

··

It happens. We get so focused on the directions to our destination, we forget to appreciate the view out the window along the way. This is true of anything we're heading toward in life: owning a house, planning a trip, saving for school. It happened to me when I was so focused on finding love, I forgot to enjoy the once-in-a-lifetime ups, downs, and bust-a-gut moments of dating. And as Gustavo and I have continued on our path toward starting a family, we make sure to tune into the other joys of life along the way.

Because one key to happiness is in recognizing that life isn't just about the "ta-da!" when you arrive at your destination, but about the moments in the middle that get you there. I love the way one character, Mr. Schuester, put it on the television show *Glee*, when the students in his glee club felt if they weren't going to win their next competition, why bother? Well, he pointed out, you bother because of the journey, because one day high school would be little more than hazy memories and forgotten names. "Life only really has one beginning and one end," said Mr. Schue, "and the rest is just a whole lot of middle."

Whether it's high school, a regular job, or the ins and outs of a daily routine, the concept is the same. Do you want to think back on this time in your life and have hazy memories of days with your head down? No. **You want to look back and have bursting, high-definition ones! So make some.** Whisk away for a weekend. Start learning Spanish like you've always wanted. Make pies. Take an acting class. Ride a bike. Ride a Ferris wheel. Learn to roll sushi. Dive in some not-warm-enough water. Fly in for a surprise party. Watch an old movie. *Make* a movie. Read a book or write one.

If you're gunning toward a goal, sit back and look at all you've accomplished so far to get there. Ask yourself: *What have I learned this past week, month, or year? Have I become smarter, stronger, and more prepared for what I'm after?* Rather than swatting away the small hurdles along your path, appreciate them. Pat yourself on the back for how far you've come and for what you're doing right now, today.

And most important, appreciate the middle of your relationships. Life isn't just about big birthdays, dance recitals, and holiday dinners; it's about the Wednesday mornings, the Sunday nights. It's the dance in the kitchen while one of you makes toast and another fills up the water pitcher; the afternoon with friends when you meet for a coffee and linger while you talk. So don't look at the renovation you started on your home as eight months of headaches, because one day you'll think back on the days in the dusty kitchen with a hot pot as magical ones. Messy maybe, but magical. And when you look at your kids, thinking, *I can't wait for the day they can fend for themselves*, remind yourself that one day you'll miss the uneventful afternoons when they needed you.

Cherish the middle moments for the fleeting times they are. Laugh, live, and learn about yourself now so you won't look back later and feel like life has passed you by. Life is a whole lot of middle. Make the most of yours.

....

Out your oughts!

....

Years ago, I was offered the job of launching a magazine and running a whole operation on my own. But hours later, walking back to my apartment, my heart started to pound, my knees started giving way, and the world blurred as I felt the rumblings of my old friend, the panic attack, knocking.

Why am I so anxious? I thought. *Because I'm nervously excited? Stunned by my good luck?* No, I realized, I was anxious because I didn't want it. But I felt I should.

"You idiot," I told my throbbing heart, "do you know how many people would kill for this opportunity? I *ought* to want it, right? I ought to grab the branch."

When I told my friend Andy about it that night, he shrugged. "Just because you *can* do something," he said, "doesn't mean you have to do it."

I exhaled in breath and spirit. Who knows if I *could* have done the job, but either way, he was right; my heart wasn't in it and that was okay. That job was someone else's dream, and I knew I'd be more motivated if I outed my "oughts" and followed my heart. So I turned down the job and chose to work for myself, where I now spend my days writing in my sunny office in Los Angeles in sight of bougainvillea blooms and butterflies, and I couldn't be happier.

When you let go of your oughts, you free yourself up to pursue your real passions. **If a choice in front of you is not in** tune with what your heart wants or how your talents are best used, it's not going to make you happier. So edge out the "ought" and follow your heart.

Author Gabriel García Márquez dropped out of his "ought" position in a Colombian law school in 1950 to write; in 1967, he published the acclaimed novel *One Hundred Years of Solitude*, and by 1982, he'd won the Nobel Prize in Literature. Britain's King Edward VIII abdicated the throne in 1936 so he could marry American divorcée Wallis Warfield Simpson, disinterested in his duties as king if he couldn't do it without the woman he loved. If he could walk away from the ought of a kingdom, you can follow what your heart wants, too.

How do you know if you're dealing with an ought? Well, an ought, essentially, is a "falsely internalized goal," explains Timothy Pychyl, PhD, a psychology professor at Carleton University in Ottawa. "Sometimes," says Pychyl, "we have to look at our goals and say, 'Why is this my goal at all?'" Maybe we're falling for what Pychyl calls "socially prescribed perfectionism." I was tempted by the falsely internalized goal of my peers—those who considered running a magazine a dream job. Once I realized it wasn't *my* goal, I was able to step away standing tall. If you find yourself saying, "I'm trying to live up to my friends' or family's expectations or the neighborhood that I live in," says Pychyl, you don't need to cave to the pressure of it. Out the oughts and be free to be yourself!

Sometimes, of course, we have to do things we don't want: We go to the funeral for our friend's dad to offer support in a time of pain, and we go to the baby showers and birthdays to celebrate the milestones. Because that's what caring partners, friends, children, and siblings do.

So how do you know if you're dealing with an ought or a "really should"? Simply ask yourself why you're doing it—find the true core in your reasoning—and you'll know. The "why" will guide you. Don't live someone else's dreams. True happiness comes by following your own.

Zoom out.

Zoom lenses can be funny things. They let you get a great close-up of a bluebird on a distant tree or a better-framed shot of a fishing boat out on the water. But have you ever forgotten to pull the zoom back in and accidentally taken a portrait of, like, someone's nostril? It's similar to what we sometimes do in life: When we find something that's grating on our nerves, we zoom in on it and miss what's going on in the whole picture. So if you feel zoomed in on a person or problem and want to fix how you feel, pull back on the lens of what you're looking at. Zoom out.

When we meet our frugal friend for lunch, for instance, sometimes all we see is how she scours for the cheapest items and mentions four times that she's "just getting the small salad" so she won't have to split the bill. When we go to a meeting at work with a complaining coworker, sometimes all we hear is how he hates his desk, his manager, and how fast cheap high-lighters start fading. **But like the camera lens of life, we can zoom out from the negative stuff and see the whole picture. Pull back and see what else is there—the *good* stuff.** You may have forgotten, but your frugal friend is also a laugh riot. And your complaining coworker is also a killer negotiator who'd give you great advice if you asked for it. So when you know you're walking into a zoom-in situation, make a conscious effort to zoom out and look at the other parts of the picture.

When I was young, we had an elderly neighbor named Madeline who was a bit crabby when we kids knocked our stickball into her yard, and who cornered us for an hour with neighborhood gossip when we picked tomatoes from our garden. Our lenses were definitely zoomed in on how she chatted away every chance she got. One year, we invited her to join us for Thanksgiving, fully prepared for her to talk until the candles on the table melted down to nubs. But wouldn't you know it, she showed up dressed in her holiday best and sat quietly with her napkin in her lap while we served up the meal. And while, true to form, she eventually did start talking, this time was different. She told stories of growing up as a coal miner's daughter in Pennsylvania, poor as a church mouse, and how her father sent her and her sisters out to walk the railroad tracks with a bucket to pick up pieces of coal that fell off the coal cars, enough to heat their house.

Hearing her life story, we couldn't help but start zooming out on Madeline. There was so much more to the picture we'd missed because we didn't try to see past one facet of her character. And the picture was touching, interesting, changing.

After that night, yeah, we sometimes still hid when she knocked on our back door to gossip. But we hid less. And we appreciated talking to her more. All it took was a reminder to zoom out. In fact, now that she's been gone for over two decades, talking about her makes me well up a little with happy memories for the large part she played in our lives.

A zoom lens is a great tool when you're focusing on something you like. But when you're seeing something you don't, pull back. Look at the other part of the picture. Intentionally focus on other traits, behaviors, or aspects of someone's personality—both the parts you know you like and the ones you just might. You may be pleasantly surprised at all you've been missing in the frame.

Write them a letter.

People are like fresh artichokes: We get the most out of them by peeling down to the heart of things. And whether we're tuning into feelings of love or forgiveness, or facing our anger, it's cathartic to pull out what's in your heart and put it onto paper in a letter.

I know, I know: You may not be the letter-writing type. You may be used to texting in short spurts and think signing a greeting card is a feat of prose, but writing down your thoughts in larger form can have powerful effects on your well-being. So if you're bursting with love, resentment, uncertainty, or regret, pull what's inside of you out in an old-fashioned letter.

When I was dumped on the street by a boyfriend years ago, I was so dumbfounded, I clammed up and crawled away. But as I replayed the scene over and over those next few days, I realized I had an opportunity to rewrite my past—or at least my emotional response to it. So I pictured myself back on that street corner, listened to his hurtful words, and began.

"Dear _____," I wrote. "How *could* you?"

Determined to preserve my heart, this time I said everything *right*. I wrote down the zingers I wished I'd used, pointed out issues I was happy to bid good riddance (he was a litterer, can you believe it?), and decided I'd be better off without him. By the time I signed that letter, I felt strong and ready to face the world again. The final step in making sure I could? I *didn't* send the letter. The fact was, having the last word—whether he knew it or not—gave me closure and strength and a lightness I hadn't felt in weeks. **That's what letters can do, lift the weight of our feelings from within us by placing them on paper.** So if you have some anger you want to get out, write it down. Whether it's been two days or twenty years since your heart was hurt, it's never too late to get off the weight.

Write a love letter, too. Make it one of forgiveness, thanks, or a heartfelt note to your spouse, your mother, your sister, or your friend. The more often you write from a place of love and appreciation, the happier you'll be and—get this—the healthier.

In one 2007 study out of Arizona State University by Kory Floyd and his colleagues Mikkelson, Hesse, and Pauley, some participants spent twenty minutes writing about someone they loved, and others about something that happened to them during the week. Five weeks later, those who had engaged in "affectionate writing"—especially writing directly *to* a loved one—were less stressed, happier, and, because their cholesterol levels had significantly dropped, healthier!

So think about it. Whether you're the "type" to write a letter or not, you'll benefit from trying. Write down why you're angry and get outrage off your chest, or write about what and who you care about and draw more love your way. However you do it, reaching down to the heart of things is a healthy way to grow.

Call it a credit in the school of life.

Gus has said that if there's one day we would have gotten divorced so far, it was on the Path of Philosophy.

Tucked at the base of the Higashiyama Mountains in Kyoto, Japan, the narrow path is just over a mile long and named after Japanese philosopher Nishida Kitaro, who used to stroll it deep in thought. There, under cherry trees and Japanese maples lit bright by the sun, Gus and I walked along the small river canal, past footbridges and benches, on our way to a famous temple at the end. It was so beautiful that as I strolled in silence behind him, I couldn't help but take photographs. Turns out, I took two hundred too many.

I learned this because when I got to the end long after he did, smiling in peace, he was already fuming. "Why did you have to stop every five minutes?" he wanted to know. "How many pictures of trees do you really need?" He was heated, I was hurting, and I worried we'd made irreparable damage in what's usually an easy-going relationship. But then the reality of it hit me: This was a crash course in each other. In every relationship, it's inevitable you'll disappoint and aggravate each other, and facing those fights head-on is the only way to learn. That day it was on a philosopher's path in Asia, tomorrow it'll be over the dishwasher in the kitchen. That's how life works: In every place, every day, we learn from our mistakes and try not to make them twice.

Consider this for your next hardship: Instead of dwelling on how pained or mad you feel over a situation gone sour, see it from another angle at the same time: **A fight, a fall, a failure, or a really rough moment in a relationship is always teaching us something. Like lessons in a classroom, look at what you've learned as one more credit toward your diploma in the school of life.**

And just like a textbook teaches us, it's often mandatory to get through tough times if we want to reach the advanced levels. Those big arguments in relationships, if you think about it, are prerequisites for intimacy. Those painful breakups are prerequisites to becoming an empathetic partner down the road. Those rough patches in your friendships are prerequisites for a bond proven to stand the ups and downs of time. Some emotional places can only be reached by learning firsthand from the teacher's podium of life.

This is true of the small things, too. One year, in a dead-end job that left me feeling like I was leveling out in learning, I started a journal I called *You Learn Something New Every Day*. At the end of every day, I wrote things like, "Learned you can tell how many minutes it is until sunset by measuring with the width of your fingers—that each finger, outstretched horizontally above the horizon, measures about fifteen minutes" or "Learned that if you cover the poked-out holes on a VCR tape with scotch tape, you can record over it again." (I, uh, started this journal a long time ago.)

Now, when I find myself in a jam that seems to have no redeeming value, I go straight to that classroom. Try it. Think: *What am I learning? What is the universe teaching me with this one?* The school of life will come through.

Those burned toast rounds? That's the school of cooking teaching you to "Set a timer." That plane cancellation? That's the school of travel teaching you to "Always confirm the flight before you leave for the airport." And if weren't for the school of shopping, you wouldn't know to check those coupon expiration dates before you head to the store.

We're not born knowing it all. In fact, we don't die knowing it all. But with all the classes that life has to offer every minute of every day, we can learn a heck of a lot along the way. Whether you're sitting behind a desk, arguing with your mechanic, or fighting your way down a quiet walking path, you're learning. Find the class credit in your next problem. And go ahead, give yourself an A.

....

Peek in your picnic basket.

....

Picture this: You're given a small basket to bring to a picnic and you can fill it with whatever sides or condiments you want. Maybe for you, it's mustard, guacamole, or a pasta salad. For me, it's a bottle of no-label, no-brand hot sauce my friend from Panama ships up every time the guy whips up a new batch. Well, what if I gave you a picnic basket for *life*? What could you bring to a situation in your life you wish was different that would make it not just palatable, but scrumptious?

Maybe it's a family relationship that's gone sour, a romance that's chilled, a job that drains your spirit. Often, we want the easy route in tough times. We want the other person or the situation to change: "I just wish my brother would stop being a selfish jerk" or "If my mother-in-law would just stop her monstrous meddling" or "If this job just wasn't so soul crushing." But **far easier than changing someone else or a situation is changing your attitude or the energy with which you come at it.** What can *you* do to change your experience for the better?

Years ago, some coworkers and I, dulled by our dreary job, created the tradition of "Taste-Off Day." Every Tuesday had a new theme—from crazy candy to bakery cupcakes to potato snacks—and we brought our best shot at winning the Taste-Off during lunch. We realized that if our work itself wasn't going to bring us the joy we wished it could, then we'd bring our *own* joy. We pulled that joy from the picnic basket in the form of hydrogenated corn syrup and sugary frosting and we were so much happier for it.

Maybe in your social life, you can be the first person to say something kind instead of laying out the groundwork for the passive-aggressive insult you feel is coming. Maybe you can swallow the pride that's been keeping you from apologizing to someone for a decade. Maybe you can ask your mother-in-law's opinion and give her a chance to feel needed before she feels the need to butt in. Or maybe, in your job, you come in an hour earlier for a month to get a jump on your projects and interact with your boss proactively instead of defensively.

Every relationship is different across families and cultures, and no one answer will work for everyone, so it's up to you to fill your own personal picnic basket. Overall, though, if something in life is leaving a bad taste in your mouth, you still have choices. You may not be able to change the physical situation, but you *can* change what you emotionally bring to the blanket. Reach into your basket for what you can bring to the table to make it better. Sometimes just a small dash of the right thing can make it the meal of your life.

Remedy the rash of regret.

I interview celebrities for magazines, which is often fascinating and sometimes challenging, but definitely different every time. I've chatted with Sheryl Crow on her couch in her living room (where she sat cross-legged and barefoot), with Kanye West at his recording studio (while he mixed "Stronger"), with Bradley Cooper at his former house in Venice (which was very modern and very clean), and with Matthew McConaughey and Kate Hudson at his trailer in Malibu (in a roomful of bongos he'd just received for his birthday). Early into my job in this genre, however, I made a mistake that makes me cringe.

I recorded a phone call with a celebrity for a small story, and because I couldn't use a backup recorder like I do in person, I also typed our conversation while we talked. An hour later, when I put my headphones on to fill in the transcription blanks, the recording sounded weird.

"Hey, how are you?" I said. "I'm so happy to chat with you!"

Then I heard . . . nothing. Just ten seconds of my fingers tapping the keyboard.

"Ha-ha-ha-haaaa, you're so funny!" I said. "Oh my God, were you dying?"

More silence. More typing.

"Uh-huh, right, right, right," I said. "Oh yeah . . ."

Silence. Typing.

"Wow. Haha, *totally*."

It turns out, instead of plugging my telephone into the microphone jack of my digital recorder, I had plugged it into the *headphone* jack. A rookie mistake. God, I still want to crawl under a rock thinking about how dumb I sounded blabbering and laughing in exchange for what *should* have been the hilarious musings of a star. I felt ill. The rash of regret was all over me. You know the feeling: It radiated from my stomach to my chest, freezing my fingertips in panic and enveloping me like a blanket I *didn't* want on.

Since there's no topical treatment for our big, fat regrets, what's the remedy? Well, you stop replaying the options of your past like a YouTube video gone viral. *(If I could do it all over, I wouldn't have picked up the phone, said what I said, left when I had . . .)* Then, you find a way to move forward. "Forgiveness," Lily Tomlin once said, "means giving up all hope for a better past." Well, you'll begin healing from regret when you forgive yourself.

Yes, it's healthy to have a postmortem of a mistake so you'll know what to do differently next time. But **there's nothing you can do about what's already happened. Like cracking the sugar on a crème brûlée, there's no going back; instead, move forward in the most positive way you can.** If there's anything you can do immediately to make your situation better, do it. Apologize to a friend, cancel the reservation, fix the order. And then . . . you deal.

Here's how I dealt with my interview catastrophe: I stopped reviewing what I *wish* I'd done, and I started brainstorming what I could do immediately to fix it. On a hunch, I rewound the tape and jacked up the sound to levels that made my voice dangerous-decibly loud and my typing sound like hammers.

And there, faintly, I could hear the star recorded through the air from my phone handset—like a pal on the couch next to you who can hear your loudmouthed friend just fine. It wasn't ideal, but I dealt, and I got the job done.

The point is, we all make mistakes. We do it in love, with

friends, with family, at work. We get caught gossiping and fibbing, sneaking in or tiptoeing out, cutting corners or making blunders. But we accept what we've done, we do what we can, we deal, and we learn from it. Since then, I've learned to double up my backups and triple-check my connections. In your own way, when you feel the regret sweeping over you, fight back the rash and run the remedy all over again.

Channel someone else's strength.

On my trip to Samoa, I met Kilisi Solomona, who told me the story of his skin-wrenching experience getting a traditional Samoan full-body tattoo. It's an awe-inspiring ritual by men who want to prove their devotion to their country and family, marking them as a public servant. But it's not for the faint of heart: The tattoo is made of ink from a burned tree nut, which is pounded into the skin by boars' tusks over twelve sessions that last five to six hours each—for three weeks.

"Right when they drew the first line in my back, I felt the pain, and that's when tears started gushing out of my eyes," said Kilisi. "The pain was unreal." After his first full day of tattooing, they cleansed his wounds in stinging salt water, batted him with palms to keep away the flies, then lay him on a straw mat on the ground. It was so difficult he wasn't sure he could carry on after the first day. "When the wind hit it, it felt like someone had peeled the skin off," he said. "Then I looked at my whole body that hadn't been done, and that's when suicide entered my mind. I thought, *There's no way I'm going to go back eleven more times. It's torture.*" But once you've begun the full-body tattoo, he says, you have to finish it, or you'll dishonor yourself and your family. Kilisi even knows men who chose suicide, who considered death an easier out.

What got Kilisi through it? "I started thinking about what my grandfather and what my family was trying to tell me," he said. "The only reason that drove me to get it done was the love for my mom. My mom is a very well-respected orator in all of Samoa. So if I couldn't get it done, her status would go down to the ground. It was only the love for my mom and my family that drove me."

When we're losing blood, we borrow another's in a miraculous transfusion of life. When the juice on our car battery is gone, we borrow a spark from someone else's. **Like a channel of water, carrying the vital elements you need, when you are all out of hope or strength, channel it from someone else.**

Kilisi's story is an example of what we'll do for family, and it's scientifically supported by a two-decades-long study published in the *British Journal of Psychology* in 2007. In it, participants endured the pain of squatting against a wall longer when they were told it would benefit family members; the closer the family bond, the longer they took the pain.

So when all you see is darkness from where you're standing, channel some strength from someone who loves you. Think how he or she would take the hurt or fear or nervousness or sadness or struggle away from you if they could and replace it with peace. Picture them placing a gift of strength within you.

Or call on family who have gone before you. When I laid down on the table for my first fertility surgery at 5:45 a.m. one chilly November morning, I pictured my nana, my gramma, my aunt Elaine, and my uncle Tommy, who had all passed away, looking down at me with pure love. And when I got a call four days later that none of our embryos were genetically healthy and the treatment was called off, I channeled strength again.

Lean on your family and friends when you need it. Whether you can see them or not, they're rooting for you, hoping as hard as you are that you make it through.

"Take a deep breath," they might say. "Now take another. I know you can do this." With their strength as yours, you will.

When
TECHNOLOGY
Is Breaking Down . . .

Reveal thyself to tech support.

My friend Todd is a hairdresser by trade and a gadget hound at heart, which means something of his is always falling apart at the chip. Well versed in the world of tech support, he knows that whether you're calling about a computer, a phone bill, a web mistake, or airline miles, trying to fix the breakdown of a product or service is the fastest way to have a breakdown yourself.

And yet, Todd almost *enjoys* calling customer service. Why? Because he's mastered having fun on the phone and looks at each call as a chance to make a boring call unique or entertain someone who's having a dull day—and he usually benefits from doing just that. He does what we could all do: Reveal thyself to tech support.

When his Internet connection was down recently, he called the cable company and said, "I had four too many drinks last night, so now I really just want to lay in bed in my underwear and watch sitcoms on Hulu all day." He laughed, she laughed, and his connection was up in three minutes flat.

Todd does this with every phone representative he calls. He'll tell his car insurance company, "I want to fix this billing issue before I head out to get a fried chicken sandwich with extra mayonnaise—because how can you have a fried chicken sandwich and *not* get it with extra mayonnaise?" And he'll tell Apple support, "I just dropped my hard drives into the toilet by accident. Just kidding! I put them there on purpose. Just kidding! Seriously, though, they're not working." If he can get them laughing—or at least thinking about something other than the drab issues they deal with all day long—he's in. **In a world that's become so automated and impersonal, getting personal is the way to get happier and get things done.** And it makes *both* of your experiences better. The reasoning is simple: "A little self-disclosure helps create closeness when you're not in the same room," explains Larry Rosen, PhD, a professor of psychology at California State University and author of *iDisorder.*

Chances are, in fact, you might not be in the same state or country, and pointing that out is another way to close an impersonal gap. "Immediately, within the first minutes, ask them, 'Where are you located, and what's the weather like?'"

suggests Rosen. "The weather is a connection everyone can make." Compared to the topic they spend all day talking about—computer glitches, phone bills, airline issues—the weather, says Rosen, "makes people soften up and they are much more helpful."

So impersonal, be darned. While others are calling tech support in bad moods about bad situations, it's a win-win to connect on a more personal, positive level. Especially if you want to wrap it up quickly so you can watch TV in *your* underwear, too.

See the grass is digitally greener, too.

Just as we think the grass might seem greener, better, and brighter on our neighbor's side of the fence, it's equally easy to fall prey to life envy online. But technology is both a powerful thing and a sneaky one: **The grass online may look greener, but for all you know, a little Photoshop editing had something to do with it.** So if you're judging your life by what you see online, it isn't a fair fight! Don't be fooled by the greenery.

The cloudless Caribbean photos your friend posted? Remember there are plenty they *didn't* show, like the view of a parking lot from their hotel window and the flies that swarmed their fish tacos. The rave reviews about a classmate's company on their site? They didn't mention they paid for that media publicity. And those chirpy Facebook posts? For all we know, they've been dealing with some tough times lately that seems too personally inappropriate to share publicly, and for now, all that feels right is to sing aloud online about the silly, lighthearted stuff instead.

Life online is like a movie trailer. People edit it to show the best parts. So while you may feel like your life seems dull or difficult in comparison to what you're reading about, it's a false comparison. When you're feeling dull compared to the divine lives of your friends online, remember: Those digital lives aren't real! So pull that imaginary green Photoshop hue tab back toward red to center it. And don't stress yourself out trying to live up to your *own* Facebook identity.

Instead, suggests Yvonne Thomas, PhD, a Los Angeles–based psychologist, ask yourself, "'What am I trying to achieve? Is it to show off? To protect an image that I'm perfect?' If you're being less than personal by being kind of phony, it's diluting the point of connecting in the first place. You've gotta be real sometimes," says Thomas, "as real as you are when you're in person or on the phone with someone. Otherwise, what's the point?"

She's right. Let's be real and stop measuring our lives by what we see online in others. The grass only looks digitally greener because it was presented that way. Your life is just as bright and fun and interesting if you choose to see it that way. Your grass is green in the right light.

Delightfully disengage.

Last month, a former classmate of mine asked me what Twitter was, as she'd never used the site to post thoughts or story links. In fact, she said, "I don't even know how to use my weefie."

"Your weefie?" I asked. "What's that?"

"You know, the Internet," she said. "In my house." Oh, the *Wi-Fi*. And while it got me laughing, I later wondered if she was onto something. I mean, there I was, logged on to *my* Wi-Fi and the work had piled up: I was writing a new blog, posting recently published material on my personal website, editing photos to upload, commenting on Facebook, and trying to keep up with those Tweets she was asking about. It was too late for me to experience the bliss of ignorance. But what about the bliss of simply ignoring my emails for an hour?

For many of us, we climb the digital Mt. Everest because it's there. But as with a mountain, just because it's there doesn't mean we have to climb it. Yes, all the videos of babies laughing on YouTube are funny, but it's also good to laugh away from the computer over a meal with friends or on a walk with your kids. **Life is like a laptop battery: It works better when you unplug it and let it run down every once in a while.** In order to appreciate what we get by being plugged in online, we have to give ourselves a chance to get free of the cord offline. Find the "off" switch and use it.

Anthropologist Genevieve Bell, Intel Fellow, former Stanford anthropology professor, and author of *Divining a Digital*

Future, told me why. "When I look at the major world cultures over the last five thousand years—like Confucianism, Hinduism, Judaism, Christianity, and Islam—every single one of them has built in downtime," said Bell. "You know, a time when you are disconnected from the materiality of the world, a time explicitly made for you to be still and quiet, or engaged in something that's not like the rest of your days. So whether it's in a separate space—whether it's dance, whether it's in song, whether it's meditation or prayer or fasting—every single world culture has this notion that you've got to change gears periodically." As human beings, Bell said, **"we need time to be disconnected from our everyday lives in order to recharge our batteries."**

To be happy, don't wait until you're overstressed about the emails building up and the digital doses you have yet to do. Build in rituals of *disconnection*. Give yourself small unplugged doses throughout your day, or build in whole days where you don't hit your "on" switch. Revel in the delight of disengaging. The "weefie" may always be on, but you deserve some time off.

Choose backward.

I was about to buy a new iPhone when I called Todd to ask which one he thought I should get. Did I need twice the memory for a hundred more dollars? He answered how I hoped he would—which, let's be honest, is why I asked.

"You won't regret getting the phone with more memory," he said, "but you *might* regret getting the one with less."

And therein lies the way my friends and I make many of our decisions: We do it backward. We base our choice not by the right now, but on how we might look back on it later. Because sometimes, mulling a choice in the moment, we're so close to it that we get consumed by the wrong details. Instead, the next time you're stressed about making a quick decision, do it backward. **Picture yourself in the future and think about what you *wish* you'd chosen. Ask yourself: What might I regret more?**

We plant our gardens backward, you know. We base the layout on what we'll wish we'd done, someday in summer's future. Will we regret planting those tiny tomato seeds two inches apart? You betcha. Instead, we give the seeds a foot or two, based on how the plants will grow and fill out and change with time—just as we will. Instead of deciding for the now, choose from the future.

Choose backward when you wonder if you should buy the fixer-upper for a killer price, or the move-in-ready remodel that might stretch you thin for years. Choose backward if you wonder if you should leave the one you're with, or if you'll regret letting them go. And if you can't decide between an obvious answer and a dark horse on a big test or a trivia game, ask which answer you might regret giving more. (For me, choosing the dark horse and hearing it was the obvious one? Ouch.) Because if it's hard to see the answer from where you're standing, moving up the block of your mind can change the perspective enough that it helps. I got the phone with more memory and with each photo and video that fills it up, I'm glad as heck I did. I didn't regret doing it, but I might have regretted *not* doing it; mistakes can be fixed and failures can be improved upon, but inaction is the seed of remorse.

Choosing backward lets you measure the "you" a few weeks or years from now and lean toward the choice of the "you" you like best. Which one will leave you lighthearted, satisfied, happy, passionate, loving, excited, and proud? Remorse is your ally when you use it as a tool for your potential happiness. Whether you're measuring computer memory, love, or the next fifty years of your life, step into the future, turn around, and choose right, right now.

Think about the postman.

I was Skyping with my friend Yvonne across the country when her cell phone rang; it was a mutual friend in another state, so she took the call, put it on speakerphone, and the three of us had a chat. Then, her cell reception failed and we both groaned.

"It's so annoying," said Yvonne. "I never get good cell reception in my apartment." It took us a minute to grasp that there we were—facing each other on our computers like a *Star Trek* future come to life—complaining that a wireless device the size of a credit card wasn't perfectly connecting in one corner of her living room.

Because, really? It wasn't that long ago that life carried on just fine without all this stuff. In 1860, American mail was delivered by the Pony Express. People wrote messages in ink on paper and a man on a horse would deliver it—a man averaging seventy-five to one hundred miles daily on a four-footed friend, and whose fastest delivery, carrying Abraham Lincoln's inaugural address from St. Joseph to Sacramento, took seven days and seventeen hours. Less than two years later, the telegraph system replaced the Pony Express, but until then, our nation survived just fine waiting a week or more for news.

Until this moment, we've been graced with the ability to connect—seamlessly, without (for me, anyway) even understanding the workings of how—in ways a nineteenth-century postman only dreamed. So the next time your connection fails, imagine the men on those horses. **Think how lucky you are that every other day this year, every minute other than these, you've been able to send the information as fast as a sneeze. Yes, you're down now, but how long have you been up!**

Without our technology, the show *can* go on. You can't email to arrange that meeting? The postman wishes a phone existed for him to pick up and call. You can't research the hotel you have to book? The postman would have loved friends so well traveled or wise to ask over lunch. You can't figure out why your camera isn't reformatting? The postman wishes he could have whisked his daguerreotype to a camera shop and ask for help.

We've become so dependent on our technological tools that

we forget how to function without them. So when technology pulls the pixel-packed rug out from under you, remember to be grateful for how well it's worked for this long, and take one step back out to the world offline to get it done.

....

Take a mental photograph.

....

We say we want to "live in the moment," but do we? As happy as I am during a fun day out, I also find myself rushing to capture it through technology—or missing the moment altogether because I'm distracted by other things. It makes me wonder: **How much of the good stuff do we lose because our minds are somewhere else, because we're not tuned into our senses at that second?** I say, put down the phone, and take a full picture with your mind, with all of your senses.

I did this for the first time one summer over dinner in the south of France with Bono. (Yes, bizarrely, that Bono.) My sister, Liz, was working for the band U2 as a massage therapist on their world tour, and I flew in to a few cities to see the shows and hang out with the gang. One night, at a small café on a sandy beach, a group of us sat for hours, drinking mojitos and talking in the warm breeze. As the moon glinted on the water we asked if someone at the table had a camera to capture it. When no one did, Bono suggested we take a mental photograph. "I taught my children how to do that," he said. "I'd tell them to take a mental picture, and then you can remember it forever." He took the lead in describing the moon over the ocean, the blue-and-white-striped cloth on the table. Someone pointed out the orchids and scent of light mint; another, the lamps and the sound of the waves.

Bono then took our hands in both of his and said, "You're in France, at the beach, in the moonlight. Make a choice to remember it forever." As if he didn't realize we already would. (Nah, Bono, we do this all the time, *bo-ring.*) But by taking turns walking ourselves through all the senses of that moment, the scene comes back to me again now—toes in the sand, the smell of the sea—in a way no photograph could have captured. And we can use this to take in the small special moments in our everyday lives, too.

Yes, photographs are great—and trust me, I take a *lot* of 'em. But when I spend a few minutes immersing myself in a moment, I feel even better. Try it: Sit in silence and take a mental photograph with all of your senses:

Ask, "What do I feel?" and work your way down your body. Feel your back, your feet, your skin warmed by the sun.

Ask, "What do I hear?" and close your eyes if it helps to focus. Maybe you hear birds, a dog barking, a friend laughing.

Ask, "What do I smell?" Breathe deeply through your nose and see what you get from this underrated sense that's so closely tied to emotion and memory.

Ask, "What do I taste?" and tune into the flavors you're drinking or eating or what's lingering on your tongue.

Ask "What do I see?" Notice the colors, the movement of things. *Who's beside you who you could be appreciating?*

We need to give ourselves the gifts of capturing these moments, being present in *this* minute of life. Not through a lens, not through a filter, not as a stepping-stone to tomorrow. Instead of using your camera to film a concert, put it away and soak the show in. Instead of texting what you see, *see* it. Instead of multitasking while you're talking to your mom, *really* talk to her and really listen. Look at what your life is giving you today—*this hour*—to be happy about and grateful for. Savor the moment. How can we really know what we want tomorrow if we don't know how we feel about today?

Let's give ourselves that gift more often than we do. The next time you find the present fleeting and life passing by, take it all in. You're here, you're healthy, in the prime of your life. Make a choice to remember it forever.

When You Hit a Bump in Your TRAVELS . . .

Put yourself in another driver's moccasins.

My sister and our friend Beth went to see a quiet film, full of striking visual scenes and very little dialogue. A few seats away, a man began whispering to his wife. Ten minutes in, Beth finally shushed them. Then the people behind the couple shushed them. Then the people in front of the couple shushed them. But the whispering went on. A half hour later, movie personnel walked in, spoke to the couple, nodded, and walked away. Yet when the whispering continued *again*, movie personnel finally asked the couple to leave.

As the pair stood up, the man turned and snapped at the room. "Blind people like to see movies, too!" he said, and walked his wife back out. Liz and Beth were stunned. All that whispering had been this kind man describing the movie, scene by scene, to his blind wife. Okay, so could they have chosen a more appropriate movie with less quiet contemplation? Certainly. But it's a lesson in how quickly we rush to assumptions about others (who woulda thunk it, right?), and how wrong we can be.

But that's what happens in public, at work, and especially on the road—be it the road of life or the street to the supermarket. We make assumptions about other people, judging their bad driving, merging, or tailgating by the four short seconds we see them in a car or movie theater. But maybe—*juuuust* maybe—we've got it wrong sometimes. And recognizing that is our first step to surviving the rage. The next time you get riled up, present yourself with a different possibility: Maybe, *just* maybe . . . there's a new way to look at it.

After all, we've been "that driver" once in a while, haven't we? I've stopped traffic trying to get out of the Right Turn Only lane I didn't mean to be in, and I've crawled my way along a street squinting at building numbers in search of my stop. Recently, I was so absorbed by a friend's great news on a phone conversation at the post office that I missed the man at the open window waving me down. *Ugh,* I thought. *I'm that girl, aren't I?* And it's just these experiences of our own we can call on to calm down our frustration with others. Psychologically, it's about practicing empathy, known figuratively as the ability to put yourself in someone else's shoes—and when we're on the road, their driving moccasins. **The way to best use your empathy is a two-step process: First, imagine your-**

self in their moccasins; second, be grateful you don't have to wear them yourself.

The guy blazing past traffic in the fire lane? Maybe he's on his way to the hospital, in a rush for the sake of his family; be grateful you're headed to work or visiting friends who'd forgive you for being late. Maybe he's had a bad day because his other half dumped him; be grateful you're having an average-to-good one and haven't just had your feelings hurt. Or maybe he's a flat-out, self-involved, narcissistic jerk; well, then, be grateful you're better than that. By putting yourself in another's shoes and imagining what life might be like for them, you give yourself the gift of forgiveness; and by looking at how lucky you are for not being in the same situation, you allow some calm back into your life.

The best gift you can give yourself in these situations is an escape route from the rage. If you can empathize and be grateful for the lane of life you're in right now, you'll be far happier along the ride.

Ask, what *didn't* you lose?

Right after college, I took a monthlong cross-country drive with a friend. Halfway through our journey, we stopped at Fisherman's Wharf in San Francisco and parked the car to get some fresh seafood and a waterside stroll. When we returned two hours later, a man knocked on our window.

"Are you missing anything?" he asked.

We shrugged, shook our heads, and began to pull out of the spot.

"Check your trunk!" he shouted through the glass.

Uh-oh. Our trunk, formerly stuffed to the nines with our tent, sleeping bags, and two duffels full of five weeks of clothes, was now empty, a hollow shell. Pale with panic, we spent three hours dealing with the cops and negotiating with the thieves to get our tent and sleeping bags back, but as for my clothes: "They liked your stuff," the messenger said. "It was all in their size."

I was angry at first, and sad every time we had another "Oh no, and my favorite *jeans!*" moment. But as we carried on toward Southern California and I bought a dress to last me the rest of the journey, I found my resentment fading. Yes, those crooks were wrong. Yet somehow, every day, I felt lighter than the last. A week later, as we headed back toward the East Coast, I felt almost invigorated owning nothing but that sundress and a sleeping bag, and I began to question my connection to all the "things" in my life at home. Did I toss out my belongings to lighten up when I returned from my trip three weeks later? Well, no. But even today when I look at all that I have, I wonder why I don't.

It reminds me of an element in the film *Up in the Air*, based on the novel by Walter Kirn. In it, George Clooney's character gives a lecture called "What's in Your Backpack?" (a spin-off of the speech "The Garage" in the novel). The larger theme of his speech is about letting go of connections with the people in our lives (to which the character's sister hilariously says, "What kind of f—ed up message is that?"). But he opens his talk by referencing all the *things* that weigh us down: the stuff on shelves and in drawers, collectibles, clothes, the television set, the kitchen table. He invites his audience to imagine putting all those items in a backpack and setting it on fire. "Let everything burn and imagine waking up tomorrow with nothing," his character says. "It's kinda exhilarating, isn't it?"

Now, don't get me wrong: When you're standing on broken glass from the smashed windows of your car, I know you'll be feeling far from exhilarated. (And you might even blame yourself—but remember, please, that someone else stealing *your* things is never your fault.) But if you find yourself reeling in your anger and you want to get over it, think about what they didn't take. What *didn't* you lose? Yeah, it's a hassle to replace phones and passports and bike seats and iPods, but the things that *really* matter? Maybe they're still with you.

Despite what's been taken or lost, maybe you still have your health or the safety of the people you love. And no matter what, you still have what's inside—that part of you that refuses to let a thief change the good you feel in your heart when you realize that what really, truly matters in life is your experience and the people around you.

That's the thing about people stealing from you: Someone else can take your things, but they can't take who you are and how you feel. And if you choose to feel grateful for all you still have, your life will feel full no matter what you've lost.

Kind of exhilarating, isn't it?

....

Plan your party story.

....

Some mornings, the alarm doesn't go off, we've run out of milk for the coffee, we get lost on the way to a meeting, and the phone battery dies before we can call for directions. In these moments, we can give up and go home, or we can see it for something else: fodder for the funniest story we'll tell all week. Because **when one thing goes wrong in a day, we've hit a bump. When three things go wrong in a day? We've got the makings of a really good story.**

When I was trying to wire money last minute through Western Union to a vacation hotel right before we left for a trip, I hit my first bump when the grocery store up the block said their system was down. I hit my second at the other place in town when they said they no longer had the service at all. When I finally found out the nearest working spot still open was forty-five minutes away, I hung up, screamed, and started banging my steering wheel like a lunatic until I noticed a mom shuffling her curious kids past my car as quickly as possible— and *that's* when I realized my experience was tipping the scales from infuriating to funny.

How do you make yourself see the future humor through the frustration you're feeling now? First, recognize that there's a level of "catastrophizing" going on, and second, visualize yourself retelling this as a laugh-out-loud cocktail yarn.

Catastrophizing is an irrational thought process that finds

the worst in a situation or, based on what's happening now, creates the worst-case scenario in your mind—far worse than it actually is in real life. But hey, when a few things go wrong in our lives at once, it's natural to lean toward it. That's when a missed flight and an overbooked hotel make you throw up your hands and say, "Our vacation is ruined! We're going to miss half the trip, end up in a grimy hotel, and waste everything we've worked so hard to plan!"

But if you step back and look down at your situation from the top of the building instead of the ground floor, you will find the view isn't as bad from up there; our problems seem less dooming when you take the Google Earth angle on it. Yes, a missed flight and canceled reservation is a major hassle, but think about this: Once you're settled in, you will feel ten times happier to be out of the airport and on vacation than you were before calamity struck. And when you get home, you have two choices: You can groan about what a nightmare mess it was, or you can build it into a funny story.

Well then, why not start building your funny story *now*? Visualize yourself next week with a rapt audience who can't believe you survived your setbacks with a smile on your face. You're not just stuck in an airport waiting room, after all . . . you're stuck with screeching teenagers on a school trip. You're not just hungry . . . you're living off of a pack of Life Savers you're rationing to the kids. And not only is your new hotel twenty minutes from the airport, you're going to have to take a local bus with no air-conditioning to get there. The worse your situation, the funnier the story. So pull back on the catastrophizing and start your story writing. Sometimes it's so bad it's good, and sometimes it's so awful it's funny. Plan your party story now and you may already start to chuckle.

Make a good scar out of it.

Matthew Moscoso is an adventure expert who helps guide snowmobiling trips with Glacier City Snowmobile Tours in Alaska. I met him during a ride into the Chugach Mountains in Girdwood, just outside of Anchorage, which is how I learned that sometimes in his world of adventure, glitches happen. Like the time Matthew was hit by an avalanche while ice climbing at the Ruth Glacier in Denali National Park, and he, his partner, and his client had to carve out a three-by-five-by-five-foot ice cave where they huddled for four days eating nothing but Snickers bars they had on hand. Sometimes, however, the slip in the plan is more subtle, like the time he took out a woman from Texas who'd bought a brand-new down puffer coat just for her trip.

As they took off snowmobiling into the woods, "a tree branch caught her new jacket as she came around the corner, putting a small tear on the shoulder," says Matthew. "She was a mess." The woman was so dampened by the downer of her new ripped coat that he sprung into action.

"Here," he said, pulling out a roll of duct tape from his knapsack. "I'll fix it." Seeing the horror on her face, he explained. "All Alaskans who've spent a good amount of time in the backcountry have duct tape or some kind of patch on their clothing," says Matthew. He pointed to his own coat, full of rips and tears, all patched up with mismatched tape from his years of war with nature. Then he pulled out a pair of scissors, cut the tape into a heart, and stuck it over the little hole. "There," he told her, "now you have a true Alaskan jacket." Her mood changed instantly, he says.

"She went from crying sadly to crying happily in two seconds! She told me she would never take it off, she loved the new patch so much. I think she liked the jacket better with the patch more so than when she bought it new!"

When life rips a hole in your perfect plan, make a scar out of it that will give you good memories to come. Sometimes, you can make it a better scar physically. You can repair the hole in your jeans with pretty fabric or an ironic-or-not Iron Maiden patch. You can wrap the knife cut around your finger with a cartoon Band-Aid. You can turn the mistake on your pottery into a unique pattern. Or you can Johnny Depp it and turn the tattoo of your ex's name into a funny phrase, the way he turned "Winona Forever" into "Wino Forever."

But whether you're able to improve upon the mistake physically or not, the key to seeing a flaw bright side up is to look at an ugly mistake in a beautiful way. That big blue ballpoint pen mark I made on my Marc Jacobs handbag? Well, that mark was made in the flurry of my busy job one weekday afternoon, before heading out to toast to the good life with my great friends. I don't work in that job anymore, or in that city, and those friends I went out with now spend quiet nights in after putting their kids to bed. That scar on my purse is a sign of a brilliant passing period of my life that I never want to forget.

Making your mark on the world is vibrant proof you've *lived* in it with some passion. See it like an "I Wuz Here" scrawl and a sign that you were moving—perhaps moving a bit too fast or a bit too shaky, but hey, you were moving. Like a duct tape heart over a rip in a brand-new coat, you can find your own way to make a good scar out of your mistakes. Let yours become a perfect life souvenir.

See it through a "look-up-to" lens.

One morning, I was driving down the street behind a girl on a Vespa scooter when the bike cut a hard left to steer around a car that had pushed its nose into the street. Because I wasn't sure if the car saw me, either, I slowed down. That's when I spotted the female driver angrily waving me on, her mouth open in glass-muted shouts behind the window, screaming, "*Goooo!* Just [bleep]ing *go* already!"

I was embarrassed to be scolded, but I sped up and carried on. Then, as the car pulled out behind me, I realized something even worse: I knew the woman. She was a *friend* of mine.

Dread set in at realizing I'd just seen this usually warm woman at her worst, probably because she was running late to work and running low on patience. To this day, I've never said a word about it, but it made me think about how we often chalk up strangers as ships passing in the night, faces in a crowd, blurs outside a window we'll never see again. When we dehumanize strangers this way, it's easier to forget our manners and forget their feelings. How else would online "haters" post mean things about what other people write, act, and say than by hiding behind their anonymity?

What if, on the other hand, when you found yourself in your less-than-ideal state of mind, you considered the thought, *Would I do that if I knew them?* Or, even more, *What if it was someone I looked up to?* Chances are you'd snap into finer form and shape up pretty fast. So how about this: **The next time you catch yourself grumbling or growling ready to roll out your worst self among strangers, imagine they're people you look up to.**

After all, we don't know there's *not* a reason to look up to them. That could be someone's aunt or mom. Someone's teacher. Someone who volunteers for charity every weekend. By seeing everyone through a look-up-to lens, you'll find yourself making the kinder, more generous choice, and feeling better about yourself for doing it.

It's funny: When I drive with the top down on our beat-up convertible, I love being the one to wave others on with a "No, go ahead, you take the turn." I've always felt it's fun gesturing in the open air above my head, but I think another part of it, honestly, is that with the roof down, I'm exposed. I'm no longer a blurred shadow behind the glass; I'm a face they can see and remember. And I don't want them to remember me as anything but gracious.

The author Hugh Prather wrote in *Notes on Love and Courage*, "Live as if everything you do will eventually be known," and I've never forgotten it. If you see others through a look-up-to lens around you, you'll be more apt to do the same. Be proud of who you are behind the steering wheel, pushing the grocery cart, standing in the discount ticket line, or dancing in the concert crowd, as if one day you will be known for it. Because someday, the person next to you *will* be someone you know and look up to. And won't you breathe a sigh of happy relief for all the practice that went into doing the right thing?

Float with the current . . . then kick to shore.

If you're ever caught in a rip current, the expert advice says: Don't fight it. Go with the flow of the water as you swim parallel to the shore until the current kicks you out and you can swim safely back to shore. The logic is, by trying to fight it, you'll tire yourself out and potentially drown, which is why rip currents cause a whopping 80 percent of surf beach lifeguard rescues. Life pulls you out on currents like that, too. And instead of wasting your energy fighting against an inevitable outcome, you're better off going with the flow, then kicking your way to solid ground you can feel good about.

My friend Mark Ellwood is a travel journalist who buys a ticket from New York to London every year to visit his parents on December 23. It's always an eight thirty a.m. flight, and it's always on British Airways and it always costs him about $900. But when he woke up the morning of his most recent flight feeling far too well rested in far too bright morning light, he knew he was in trouble. It was the age-old mistake: He'd set his alarm for six *p.m.* instead of six a.m. and missed his flight.

When he called the airline in a panic, they said, essentially, "No worries, we'll get you another seat. In fact, yes, here's one on a later flight for a slight change fee that brings your ticket up to . . . ah, yes, there it is: just over two thousand dollars for a few days with Mum."

Mark begged for a way to fix it, but the more he tried fighting it, the more he realized it was for naught—especially because it was his mistake in the first place. So he took a new tack: Mark let the current take him and his credit card for the ride, and as soon as he got to the airport, he pleaded his way into a Business Class seat for the same price and spent the long flight drinking free wine and falling comfortably asleep on a fully laid-out bed, so by the time he got to Mum, he was well rested and happy to be home.

When Mark first told me that story, I was waiting for a happier ending. "Wait," I said, "so you still had to pay the extra thousand bucks?" He had to remind me his happy ending wasn't in the money he was or wasn't saving—it was in how he *felt* about his situation. Mark made his own happy ending by recognizing what he would never be able to control—the price of his seat—and changing what he could by getting the best seat he could for the price. It was the ultimate lesson in seeing bright side up. Like the "serenity prayer" attributed to theologian Reinhold Niebuhr in the first half of the twentieth century, it is calming to **accept the things we cannot change and change the things we can. In other words, float with the current and then kick your way to shore.**

When the department store is adamant they'll only issue a store credit, or you're reassigned at work, or your flight is delayed, don't fight the inevitable outcome. If you can't change a store policy or a boss's mind or Greenwich Mean Time across the continents, go with the flow—then make the most of the place you're in.

You never know. Maybe the department store credit can buy a friend a birthday present, a work project teaches you a new skill set, and missing your alarm like Mark did means you get to drive to work on traffic-free streets with your windows down on a sunny day. Don't waste your energy fighting pointless battles. Go with the currents you can't change, then make the most of what you can.

There is beauty. Take it in.

Sit two people in front of the same pond and they may see different things. One might see a serene spot where baby ducks come to play; the other, stale water, mosquitoes, and grass you don't want to sit on without a thick blanket. Two people can see a crowd differently, too: One might see the energy of like-minded people coming together; the other, sweaty strangers and a hellish commute home. In a scene in the 1999 film *American Beauty*, the character Ricky shows some video footage he took of the beauty of a plastic bag, floating on uncertain wisps of the wind—a bag that, from another point of view, can also pass for plain garbage littering the sidewalk. **There are always two opposite ways to see things. And in one of those ways, there is beauty. Take it in.**

On a crowded city street, plagued by a cacophony of horns, brakes, and whistles for cabs, perhaps there is beauty in the elderly woman plotting a path along the sidewalk with her walker in measured determination or in the one tree standing proud over it all. Or maybe there's beauty in the reflection of the clouds on an office building window, floating slowly from one mirrored slice to another. In a traffic jam, among the humming of bored engines, perhaps there is beauty in the flowering weeds fighting through the freeway's cement divide, or in the dog in a window, panting happy breath against the glass, or in the hills in the distance, lit just so by the sun.

In the mirror in the morning, there is beauty in a face that's all your own. I don't always love the bump on my nose, but I got it from my mom and nana, and it's a gift of our unique family history passed along in my own features. And when I'm not loving the way my body looks, I need only look back at photos from ten years ago when I wasn't loving the way my body looked then, either. *What, was I crazy?* I'll think. *I looked great back then!* Well, it's safe to say that in ten years, I'll look back at myself and think I looked pretty great right now, too, so why wait ten years to see the beauty in the body I have? It's far much more fun to appreciate it today.

When you are caught in what feels like a place of ugly—in your surroundings or how you feel about yourself—shift what you're looking at and flip what's in front of you. Life is beautiful. Take it in.

Let them pass.

I'm not a big fan of the airport baggage claim. And my recent experience reminded me why. I'd gotten myself a nice spot two feet back from the edge of the carousel where all of us passengers could see and reach the bags approaching. Then a big, burly guy pushed his way past us and posted up against the carousel.

Well, now we couldn't see around the guy to our bags, and when some people stepped up beside him and *he* couldn't see past *them* to the bags, he began "the lean." You know the one: Once he leaned forward over the carousel, each successive person did, too, until an entire row of passengers were bent over, balancing on their tippy toes.

Sigh, I thought. *We had it all worked out, people! If we all stood two feet back, we could all see our bags.* Now, it was a mess. And at six thirty a.m., far too early for one. So I took a deep breath, stepped back, and walked to the other side. It's a tactic that helps me shed my frustration faster than any other: **Quietly thank a stranger for the life skill they're letting you practice, then step back and let them pass.**

When you think about it, every frustrating act of a stranger offers us some test of our kinder, better human qualities. The man at the baggage claim tested my patience. A person hogging your armrest tests your selflessness about your personal space. A woman who starts another line in an already-efficient one-line system at CVS tests your tolerance, compassion, flexibility, and ability to forgive.

But either way, the next step is to stand back and let them pass. *Let them pass?* you might think. *And let them get the armrest? The spot in front? The next place in line?* Well, the way I see it, you can spend your time focused on the nerve of some people, or you can give it up and enjoy the ride. When a car is tailgating me on a one-lane road, it tests both my patience and my pride—Should I keep steady and ignore them? Slow down to spite them?—but I've found neither choice makes me feel as happy as pulling over, letting them pass, and then continuing on my way. Would I like to see them pulled over for speeding four miles later? Ooh, I'd love that. But I love more that I was able to let it go and enjoy my drive stress-free. The same thing works in the movies. Now, when someone in a theater is talking behind me, instead of signing up to turn and shush them for two hours, I get up and move to another seat.

Give your boiling point a break sometimes. Don't let the

nagging habits of strangers eat away at your day. Find a way to thank them for the lesson you're getting in life, then step back and let them pass. Life in your lane is more pleasant when you do.

Find your piña colada.

My husband likes to say a vacation doesn't officially start until we've had a piña colada. There's something so magical about holding the icy glass in our hands, smelling that coconut, and taking a bite from that slice of pineapple that sets off memory receptors of relaxation and vacation. The same way Russian physiologist Ivan Pavlov famously trained his dogs to salivate for dinner upon hearing a bell ring, we can become conditioned to feel relaxed and calm the minute we smell, taste, or sense vacation moments in our everyday lives.

You may not like piña coladas, but you must have something that feels like vacation, too. Is it curling up with a good book? Lingering over a cup of coffee? Riding a bike? Putting on fuzzy socks? **Identify what turns on your "vacation" switch—your version of a piña colada—and bring that relaxing fun into your everyday life.**

Here at home, for instance, when I really need to decompress, I've found that bringing island scents into my life makes me feel more relaxed. I bought an Alba gardenia shampoo that smells like the tropics, some beachy-smelling "Shore" hand soap from Restoration Hardware, and candles that smell like coconuts to light when I really want to chill out. And sometimes, after a tough week, Gus and I will hit a place up the road and order piña coladas as a "staycation" way to unwind. After all, most of us aren't getting much actual vacation time; although most Americans receive about two weeks of paid vacation—versus thirty or more days in countries like France and Finland—many of us don't even take all the days we're allotted. And we may not be able to afford visiting paradise when we do. So find a way to bring vacation to you.

If you spend a lot of time reading business journals or textbooks, decompress with a good mystery or romance novel every once in a while. If you spend a lot of time making meals for your family, go out for a big pancake breakfast one weekend morning like you only do when you're out of town. And if you're caught up in the routine of a relationship or you're dating so much the nights are blending into one, find your piña colada in love. What makes you feel like you can exhale and truly relax in the presence of the person you're with? Is it walking through a park, eating ice cream, playing Skee-Ball? Maybe you can't help falling in lust again if you hole up in a fancy hotel room.

Life's too short to save the special stuff for one or two weeks a year. Make your own piña colada and relax into a little vacation with your first sip.

Enjoy the right-this-second now.

I'm not always kind to my right-this-second self. On the train, sometimes I don't take off my coat and hang it because I'll just have to put it back on later. I don't open a newspaper for a subway ride because then I'll have to fold it back up. To this day, even, I'll put my airport carry-on bag under the seat in front of me instead of in the overheard bin in case I have to get something out of it later. But often, the only "thing" I get out of it is a leg cramp from trying to get comfortable around it. Instead of enjoying my right-this-second, I defer happiness to my future self.

Author Hugh Prather recognized a similar trait in himself in his 1972 book, *I Touch the Earth, the Earth Touches Me*: "Not opening a can of tuna because last night's roast will spoil if I don't eat it," he wrote. "Not changing the thermostat because later it might get too hot; not pulling over the coffee table to eat on because I will have to put it back—I am surprised at how much I indenture myself to the future." Are you also putting off enjoying your right-this-second to make it easier for you in an hour?

Maybe you're not lighting a candle you love because then you'll have to buy another one. Or you're not making cupcakes because you don't want to clean up after them later. Or you're not going out on dates because you might not have time to devote to a relationship anyway. Or you turn down the cup of hot tea from the Thai take-out joint because waiting five minutes for your food isn't long enough to enjoy tea, is it? Until

I wrote this very chapter, Gus and I still showered in a plain white bathroom we never bothered to paint because someday, we figured, we'd just have to paint it back again. Now, it's a soothing shade of silver sage, and I wonder why it took me five years to give ourselves that gift.

Hey, sometimes the things we do today—eating well, working out, practicing guitar—are beneficial for our future selves. **But if you're sacrificing the happy you this second only because you don't think a small enjoyment is worth it, you're missing out. From now on, let yourself enjoy the right-this-second!**

Paint the bathroom. Light the candle. Make the cupcakes *with* the crunchy nonpareils that might spill all over the kitchen floor. Enjoy the right-this-second every single day. Your future self ten minutes from now will be pretty happy you did.

Leave the "should haves" at the door.

My sister went on a weekend canoe trip down the Batsto River in New Jersey. After loading tents, fire supplies, and food into two canoes, she and her friends paddled downstream. An hour later, their friend Jurg began searching the hull of the boat for his camera bag.

"Has anyone seen my camera bag?" he asked frantically.

My sister and her friends looked at each other with shock,

then guilt, for each one of them, independent of the other, knew just where it was: his bright red camera bag was still sitting on the side of the shore. "We were all so certain someone else would grab it," Liz says, "that none of us said anything." My sister and her friend Jennifer kicked themselves. Because not doing what they "should have" done was now costing them time and the guys some serious paddling effort. This happened a few more times—when some wondered later if they "should have" set the tent up in a different spot, or "should have" put the matches in the plastic bag overnight, so they made a rule based on "the Batsto Phenomenon": "If you think it, there's no good reason *not* to say it." Now, my sister is always the one to say when we're leaving a restaurant, "I know this seems obvious, but you're going to grab your jacket over there, right?" (And until she'd said so, no, I wasn't.) They handled their "should haves" well and we can all gain from doing the same.

Like a pair of muddy boots you leave on a front mat before you enter the room, leave your "should haves" behind, too. **Instead of sulking in the depths of should haves, would haves, and could haves, make your new mantra this: "I *should* have, but I *didn't*, so what *can* I do now?"**

You can use this in so many situations: When your car is broken into and you realize you "should have" put your messenger bag in the trunk out of view. Or when you take the train ten stops the wrong way and see you "should have" asked someone on the platform before you got on. Okay, sure, maybe you *should* have done those things, but you *didn't*, so what *can* you do now? Think of this the next time you want to beat yourself up. So you didn't bring new batteries for the flashlight. So you didn't start investing into your retirement account ten years ago. So you didn't tell the guy or girl you just went on a date with that you'd love to seem them again. So you didn't back up your digital photographs on an external hard drive. *It happens.*

"Should haves" have no place in productivity; they do nothing but slow down your forward movement and distract your mind, so leave yours at the front door. And, like my sister's Batsto Phenomenon, say what seems obvious, tell your dates how you feel, load up on gas, leave word with a loved one before a trip, and for the sake of your sanity, back up your computer files! Make your next "should have" count for something. Say: "I *should* have, but I *didn't*, so what *can* I do now?" and then chalk up all that "should have" learning so your future self *can*.

The good news is . . .

After something goes wrong in your day, you can almost picture the headline:

GUY PARKS IN STUPID SPOT, GETS CAR TOWED

COUPLE WAKES UP NEIGHBORHOOD WHILE SCREAMING ABOUT STOVE

CLUMSY GIRL KNOCKS DRINK ALL OVER TABLE

But if you challenge yourself to find "the good news" about an un-good thing, you might get yourself laughing your way out of it.

Yes, your car just got towed. The good news is . . . you've always wondered what that neighborhood around the tow lot looked like, and now you'll get to find out. Yes, you and your partner had a loud fight. The good news is . . . the raccoons have been scared away from your house for a while. And yes, you just spilled your entire margarita on the table. The good news is . . . there's more where that came from and it's only four feet away.

Use your imagination: Start with the practical and go to the preposterous. Just say, "Well, the *good* news is . . ." and like a game of Boggle where the person who finds the most words among the letters wins, the more "good news" you can come up with about your situation, the more you win. **We may not see much good news in and on the news, but in our own lives, *we're* the reporters and we make the headlines.**

Gus and I had just had the best zip-line experience of our lives at Sky Trek at Monteverde, Costa Rica, when we hit a glitch: Our 4x4 got a flat tire—at dusk, in the rain, while it was thundering and lightning. And as we talked about it over dinner, all we kept coming back to was how lucky we were. Why? Well, the good news was we got our flat in a wide-open parking lot instead of on a hill or on a curve on a dirt road. The good news was two guys just leaving work helped us change it and one of them led us to a local mechanic in town. The good news was we got to the shop five minutes before it closed and had enough cash to pay to get it done. So yeah, we got a flat tire in a thunderstorm, but man, were we lucky. Unlike the stuff that comes in the paper, news isn't always black and white. So take the gray and spin it into something brighter.

Yes, you have the flu; the good news is . . . you'll get to catch up on your Netflix viewing. Yes, your boyfriend dumped you; the good news is . . . you'll get to indulge in the Indian food he never wanted to have. Sometimes, the worse the bad news, the more fun it is to find some far-fetched good news about it.

You can even carry this trick into your daily routine, through the "three good things" exercise developed by Christopher Peterson, PhD, professor of psychology at the University of Michigan; Martin Seligman, PhD; and their colleagues Park and Steen. As they suggest, after dinner and before bed, write down three things that went well during the day, and then answer the question, "Why did this good thing happen?" The results are effective: "We found that counting one's blessings increases happiness and decreases symptoms of depression for up to six months of follow-up," writes Peterson in *A Primer in Positive Psychology*. And, he adds, "sixty percent of the participants in the study reported that they were still counting their blessings six months later."

Feature the good news and you will find it. Yes, it takes work to find pearls in a junk pile. The good news is . . . you're clever enough to pull it off.

EPILOGUE

Look on the BRIGHT SIDE...

Life simply seems better when you can view it from a more positive perspective.

The next time you run out of gas, gain ten pounds, freeze up your computer, break your favorite glass, or get dumped, bruised, insulted, or let go, maybe one of these hundred ideas can help shift your standpoint just enough.

Remember, you don't have to change who you are, where you live, what you wear, and how much money you make to have a happier life. For **one key to a happy life is in benefiting from what you already *have*. If you want to be happy, look at things bright side up.** Wear your heart on your sleeve and dress from the inside out. Keep your eyes on your prize, then trust the path, as far off course as it's leading you. Seek a smiler on the street, seek the strengths within yourself, and see how lucky you are that at least you're not in a place that, really, could be worse. Don't let fear hold you back from trying something brave, for taking a chance is success in itself. Stop beating yourself up and stop aiming for perfect, because the crooked, gloppy cinnamon buns of life always taste just as good. Try new things and appreciate the old. And if you fall on your face in front of the room, stand up, laugh it off, and create your own tone of confidence for what's to come. Your life is art; you—with all your bumps, freckles, and bad punch lines—deserve a luminous life. Allow it in. Rise to the level you're capable of. Let your every day shine.

Your life is what you make of it and your experience is how you see it. And there are endless ways to view what's right in front of you from another angle. I work on doing this every single day, which is why, although Gus and I still haven't had luck on the baby front, the good news is . . . we're happier than ever together, and I've chosen to look at the time we have, just the two of us, as a precious gift. I know that whatever life brings us from here on out, we'll make the most of it. Maybe we'll have a family or continue to *be* each other's family in the great adventure of life. Either way, we'll be happy. I don't want to spend these dear days of my life wanting. Because a truly happy life isn't about what we'll get or be tomorrow, it's about feeling grateful for our abundance today.

Let's not spend our days striving and trying with an "if . . . then" life. You know: *If* we get the job or house or wife or couch, *then* we'll be happy. Because the "if . . . then" formula doesn't lead to happiness the way appreciating our experience today *can*. Start looking at what you have right now from a perspective that lets the bright side in. Appreciate the Thursday afternoons, the routine drives, the blueberries in season, the shorthand you use to communicate with family, and the contentment on the faces of those you love. When you look at what you have from a fresh, positive place, you can feel happier in your own shoes without changing a thing.

In fact, you probably have your own bright-side-up strategies that help you do just that. Tell me: What's worked for you? How did you turn a tough experience into a positive one? I'd love to know. Share what you've tried and what works at www.brightsideup.com. And if you find yourself in a particular pickle and need help seeing it from a happier place, go to the reference guide online at www.brightsideup.com/turntoguide to find the point of view that might work best.

The magic of happiness is in how we view the hand we're dealt. The brighter it looks, the better.

ACKNOWLEDGMENTS

I want to first thank my agent, Laurie Abkemeier, for her brains, warmth, humor, and for somehow seeming to work thirty-four hours a day and making me feel like I'm the only writer in her life. People told me not every agent will hold your hand and encourage you. Well, lucky me, mine does.

And I want to give big thanks to Marian Lizzi, my editor at Perigee, for believing in this project. Before we worked together, I heard more times than I can count, "Aw, man, you get to work with Marian?" They were right. I've felt safe and inspired every step of the way. Thank you, Nellys Liang and Tiffany Estreicher, for the charming design; Erin Galloway, for getting the word out; and the whole Perigee team who made this book a beautiful reality.

I want to thank all of the experts I spoke to for the book, for having your insights meant the world. And to those who let me include your good, bad, and embarrassing tales, thank you. It's through the trials of life that we learn—but it's sure easier when it's *other* people's trials we get to learn from.

Thank you to all my Twitter followers, my Facebook pals, all TheLifeOptimist.com readers, and my "Vitamin Optimism" newsletter members. (If you're not signed up to get the happiest email you'll get all week, go to www.brightsideup.com and get on board!) It warms my heart to communicate and connect with all of you, all over the world.

A big thank-you to my close friends, who supported me as I brainstormed, wrote, revised, and essentially didn't stop talking about the book for a year, and who contributed in vast ways just by being them: Todd Bush gets my deep-fried love for being there, always. So do Yvonne Cheoun; Phillip Graybill; my "Dolphinitas" Patty Bilotti, Jenn Gardiner, and Kerry Cushman; Brandon Young; Beth "the Vortex" Greenwald; Courtney Freeman; Mike Verna; and Johnny White. Eric Gordon gets a high five for being a rare breed of "web guy" who does things really dang well, and with laughs along the way. I also want to give a shout-out to Dr. Sepilian, Tina, and Diana, for whatever happens, you've softened the road like friends along a really tough ride.

Thank you to my mom, Katherine Spencer, and my dad, Ken Spencer, for your help, suggestions, and, of course, for the whole "loving me" thing. And thank you to my sister, Elizabeth Spencer, for supporting me, for taking the stress knots out of my neck with your master massages, and for being four blocks away and—literally—here when I need you.

I also want to thank my other mother, Silvia, and my other sister, Mariana, for being the best in-laws a girl could ask for. It doesn't seem fair I get a second family as wonderful as you! And to the rest of my family, thank you for your love and eternal support: JoAnne, Vincent, Patrick, Christopher, Bethany, Angela, and Finley; Joan, Karen, Betsey, Jonathan, Jenny, Lauren, Kelsey, and Chris; Neil, Tracy, Maureen, Bill, Bob, Brett, Karen, Todd, Jenny, Brendan, Jeff, Kelly, Connor, Katie, Nicki, Keera, Jessica, and Lauren; Martha, Raul, Santiago, Carolina, Jen, Arthur, and the family in Argentina; and those who have passed along ahead of us. I've learned from and been made better by you all.

My warmest thanks go to Gustavo, my husband. He read drafts of the book more than anyone who didn't write it should have to, patiently offering his opinion and some great ideas. (Oh, see, he suggests I change that to "divinely inspired" ones. I'll give it to him.) He also manages to bolster the both of us when the optimist in me is out to a long lunch and just wants to come home and nap. For all that you are and all that you do, thank you.

As for Tarzan and Guinness, thanks for the purrs and nuzzles when I needed them, but I'll thank you guys with tuna sashimi, which I'm sure will mean much more.

And thank *you* for reading this book—all the way down to here! If you guessed you were getting a big figurative hug, you were right. Thank you. For without the hope of you reading this book, I wouldn't have been able to write it. And I really wanted to write it, to play a part in getting as many people as possible to see the positive parts of the lives we all have right now. If my ideas can help shift your view in just one situation on one crummy day, I will be happy. So please, let me know if they have at amy@amyspencer.com. Because I like being happy. And I want the same for you.

ABOUT THE AUTHOR

Amy Spencer is a Los Angeles–based journalist, relationship expert, and life optimist. She is the author of *Meeting Your Half-Orange: An Utterly Upbeat Guide to Using Dating Optimism to Find Your Perfect Match* and has written for *Glamour, Harper's Bazaar, Real Simple*, CNN.com, and others. Amy has appeared as an expert on NBC, CBS, VH1, and Fox News. She loves cooking shows, biking, paddle tennis, and traveling, and she loves popcorn so much, she rolled a popcorn cart right into her living room. Amy lives with her husband in Venice, California. Visit her website at www.amyspencer.com.